INCREDIBLE EDIBLE

Gluten-Free Food for Kids

150 FAMILY-TESTED RECIPES

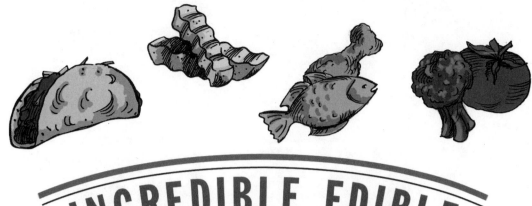

INCREDIBLE EDIBLE

Gluten-Free Food for Kids

150 FAMILY-TESTED RECIPES

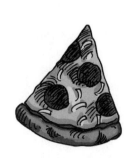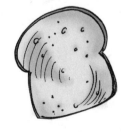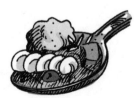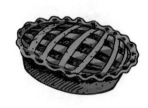

Sheri L. Sanderson

Woodbine House ■ 2002

All rights reserved. Published in the United States of America by Woodbine House, 6510 Bells Mill Road, Bethesda, MD 20817.
www.woodbinehouse.com

Cover design and all illustrations by Linda Lampman, with the exception of iceberg graphic on page 13, which is courtesy of Dr. Karoly Horvath, Center for Celiac Research, University of Maryland Medical School.

Library of Congress Cataloging-in-Publication Data

Sanderson, Sheri L.
      Incredible edible gluten-free food for kids : 150 family-tested recipes / by Sheri L. Sanderson.—1st ed.
          p. cm.
      Includes index.
      ISBN 1-890627-28-3 (pbk.)
       1.Celiac disease—Diet therapy. 2. Gluten-free diet—Recipes. 3. Gluten-free diet. I. Title.

RC862.C44 S26 2002
641.5'638—dc21

                                                                                            2002023496

Manufactured in the United States of America
First edition

10   9   8   7   6   5   4   3   2   1

"A hundred years from now . . . it will not matter what my bank account was, the sort of house I lived in, or the kind of car I drove . . . but the world may be different because I was important in the life of a child."
—Kathy Davis

This book is dedicated, first and foremost, to God, who inspired it, provided the courage and strength to accomplish it, and answered my prayers for resources and for ideas.

It is also dedicated to my family:
To my husband, Rob, for not questioning the dream and supporting me, to my son, James, whose need prompted the book, and to my other children, Linda and Aaron, who patiently tested my recipes and endured my culinary failures.

I love you all!

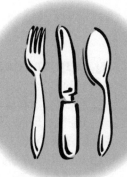

Table of Contents

Acknowledgements

"Those who have a 'why' to live can bear with almost any 'how.'"
—Frank Victor

This cookbook is not only a collection of recipes, but also a collection of experiences. I owe a debt of gratitude to many people:

To Cynthia Kupper, RD, CD, Executive Director of the Gluten Intolerance Group, for educating me on various aspects of celiac disease and gluten intolerance as I struggled to help my son regain his health.

To Bette Hagman for being my mentor, guiding me through the correct way of writing a cookbook and the ins and outs of developing recipes, and for her friendship.

To my illustrator, Linda Lampman, for her beautifully made illustrations from my atrocious sketches, her super-positive attitude, and her willingness to help me.

To Susan Stokes and the staff of Woodbine House for their hard work and for making this writing experience so positive for me.

To Dr. Alessio Fasano and Dr. Karoly Horvath of the Center for Celiac Research at the University of Maryland for their dedication to celiac research and for allowing me to reap many benefits of their research.

My appreciation goes out to Sam Wylde III of Ener-G Foods for help with technical questions, support, and friendship; Eva at the front desk of Ener-G Foods for sending prospective testers my way; Steve Rice of Authentic Foods for ideas, support, and sending potential testers my brochures with their orders; and Jay Berger of Miss Roben's for the use of her extensive troubleshooting guide.

Professional advisors I am graciously indebted to include: Dr. William Graf, Dr. Brian Vlcek, Dr. Kenneth Fine, Dr. Thomas Self, and Dr. Louie G. Linnerelli.

For her love and support, I thank my close friend Marcia MacHaffie, a fellow celiac who suspected a wheat intolerance months earlier than anyone else. I thank my friends, Sam Brumit, Joyce Lynch, and Barbara Kellenbarger, for their support, and June Stokes for moral support and prayer.

And, of course, thank you to the families who tested these recipes and ideas to help make this a guidebook instead of just another collection of recipes:

Jennifer Abernethy
Janet Adamek
Rose Barry
Lynda Benkofske
Mimi Blank
Howard Boksenbaum
Tanya Buchwald
Cindy Bucy
Jill Canales
Mary Carson
Christine Chernjavsky
Tanis Collard
Kim Cordner
Jenny Cronin
Lynessa Cronn
Cindy Cummins
Kenneth Fine, M.D.
Melissa Garden
Sharon Hockenbury
Lillian Horn
Jennifer Hall Jones
Frances Kelley
Danna Korn
Susan Lair
Sandy Lepire
Judith Liran
Sue Loseke
Marcia MacHaffie
Kay Meadows
Rebecca Meinert
Phyllis Millay

Kerrie Newton
Wendy Percival
Lori Ratajczak
Steven J. Rice
Lori Ross
Susan Ross
Linda Smith
Jessica South
Ann Srdar
Melissa St. Clair
Leigh Sutherland
Nancy Uding
Millie van Eerde
Mildred Walton
Tracey Wolfskill
Jean Young

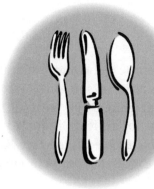

Foreword

By Cynthia Kupper, RD, CD
Executive Director of the Gluten Intolerance Group™

Often parents are relieved to find out what is wrong when their child is first diagnosed with a gluten intolerance. They know their child will live and be healthy again. Later, they and their children may begin to see the gluten-free diet as an insurmountable mountain of "can't haves" and "not alloweds." Although the restrictions of the diet may seem unattainable to you if your child has just been diagnosed, they really are not. It's all in how you look at it and how you teach your child to look at it.

A well-rounded gluten-free diet, with a lot of variety, is able to provide all the nutrients a child needs. Just as importantly, studies show that early detection of gluten intolerance in children may spare them from the problems related to malnutrition that are often seen in people who are not diagnosed until adulthood. Children are able to grow normally and have fewer behavior and learning problems when they are absorbing all the nutrients they need.

Gluten-free foods are so good these days that many people would never know they were eating a gluten-free cookie or pizza. However, because children may take time getting used to the new textures and tastes of gluten-free foods, it may be a good idea for your child to take a daily vitamin supplement. Be aware, too, that it is not unusual for children to go on eating jags (eating only a select few items for long periods of time). Concentrate on teaching your child to try new foods and tastes, eat some fruits and vegetables every day, and get a good source of protein for growth. Don't eliminate sweets and "junk" foods. Instead, teach your child to make other choices and learn to limit high fat or high sugar foods. Variety is the spice of life, and learning to exercise self-control with high caloric foods will help your child control weight issues as he or she grows into an adult.

When children learn to eat gluten-free early in life, and the experience is positive, the adjustment is really not difficult. It quickly becomes just one part of a healthy, happy lifestyle. *Incredible Edible Gluten-Free Food for Kids* can help show you how to create that positive experience for your child.

Introduction

"The distance doesn't matter; it is only the first step that is difficult."
—Marquise du Deffand

Imagine a childhood without birthday cakes, hot dogs, apple pie, spaghetti, pizza, or macaroni and cheese. Life for a child with gluten intolerance can seem hopelessly restrictive. Preparing meals for that child can be incredibly overwhelming for the parents and caregivers—at least, in the beginning. But living without wheat or gluten should not condemn a child to living without tasty, nutritious, and fun foods!

This book provides recipes for tasty, nutritious, fun kid foods that most of us have taken for granted. Serving your child these kinds of foods is important, because no child wants to eat things that make him feel out of place at school, at a friend's home, or at a birthday party. Although wheat or gluten products must be removed from the diet for your child's health, this does not mean that he can no longer enjoy food!

The recipes in this book have been tested in the homes of over fifty children with celiac disease or wheat/gluten intolerance. This means other parents and caregivers, just like you, have helped to create a book that will assist your child through those years when adult foods seem "yucky."

The goal of this book is to cater to the young child's palate. It is my hope and prayer that you and your family will see improvement in your gluten-intolerant child(ren) with the use of this book.

Personal Beginnings

"I know God will not give me anything I can't handle.
I just wish that He didn't trust me so much."
—Mother Teresa

"Just for giggles, take your son off wheat," said the doctor of the Neurodevelopmental Clinic, where I had brought my son due to his failure to thrive and constant diarrhea.

"Well, great. Now what?" Armed with a list of ingredients to avoid from the hospital's nutritionist, I headed to the grocery store. Two hours later, I came home with "corn pops," corn tortillas, and rice cakes! Surely my son would starve on this diet! (Sound familiar?)

My son grew normally for the first six months, despite having been born with clubbed feet. (He had casts on his feet coming home from the hospital.) At six months, around the time I introduced solid foods, James began arching his back and throwing tantrums. He had many "colds" with an upset tummy. James became quite constipated at eight to nine months. I did as any mother would and increased fruits such as prunes to help things along. At nine months of age, he had corrective surgery on his feet, a four-and-a-half-hour procedure. The surgeon reported to us during a break between working on his feet. I remember him telling us, "This child has pooped the entire time we've been in surgery. What have you been feeding him?" We laughed about it at the time, but looking back, it was only the beginning of his symptoms.

When James was between nine months and a year old, we began to notice poor weight gain. His pediatrician told me to increase solids to expand his stomach capacity. He began eating even more solid foods, but his health continued to decline. At fifteen months, James was seen for a recheck of his "diarrhea illness" that had been off/on for one and a half weeks. He had been placed on the BRAT diet during that time (B – banana, R – rice, A – applesauce, T – toast). The doctor's notes indicated, "Diarrhea illness, resolving. Mom is to gradually advance his diet. … If he is not back to normal over the next week, she is to let me know. I feel with more solid food he should increase his stomach capacity and his stools should start to firm up."

At James' two-year check-up, his pediatrician noted new concerns: "Poor weight gain, short stature, concern over possible speech delay." At this age, James was also beginning to bang his head. We tried to ignore it, but the head banging continued.

In addition, he was pulling hair, biting, and engaging in other behavioral concerns. He was also anemic (low iron in blood levels).

When he was two and a half, James weighed as much as the average twelve-month-old child. He was well below the fifth percentile in both weight and height—even though he had a large appetite and ate three meals a day plus two snacks, all high calorie foods. He took a multi-vitamin with iron, yet still had anemia. James had ongoing behavioral concerns with head-banging and throwing tantrums. The pediatrician also noted a concern of a developmental delay, especially in speech. At this appointment, many lab tests were ordered. The notes read, "Depending on the results of [the laboratory] studies, consider further evaluation for milk intolerance or allergy or possible celiac disease."

James was tested for allergies. His report stated, "No evidence of true food allergies or IgE antibody [required antibody for allergy testing to work], may have food intolerance."

When James was thirty-seven months old, we received the "just-for-giggles" diagnosis. And although he survived his first week on the gluten-free diet (mostly on Corn Pops® and corn tortillas with melted cheese), the diet seemed so dull and unappetizing. I bought every gluten-free cookbook I could find—cookbooks written for adults by authors such as Bette Hagman, Carol Fenster, and Jax Peters Lowell, to name a few. My husband and I enjoyed many of the recipes, but my kids wouldn't eat them. I was overwhelmed as I tried to find "kid" food for my son. In vain, I looked and looked for cookbooks written to appeal to a child's tastes, yet without wheat or gluten. So I began to convert my family's favorite recipes to fit within the gluten-free diet guidelines.

Within three months of starting on the gluten-free diet, James' diarrhea had become pasty instead of watery, he had slowly begun to gain a little weight. His speech improved from the level of an average eighteen-month-old to that of an average twenty-nine-month-old in the same three months. On the gluten-free diet, his improvements in health, speech, and behavior were amazing!

One day, a friend with a wheat-allergic son stopped by for lunch and I served my gluten-free pizza. They both loved it! My friend asked where I had found the recipe and I told her I had developed it. "You ought to write a cookbook just for kids," she suggested. The idea for this book was born.

James has been on the gluten-free diet since November 1997. By October 2000, his gut had finally healed enough that his body was able to resume growing at a consistent rate, but his behaviors were still a concern. He was diagnosed with obsessive-compulsive disorder (OCD) at nearly four years old. An additional diagnosis of high functioning autism followed when he was five and a half. He began taking medications and he entered into a special day class. He has made significant improvements with the gluten-free diet, medication, and interventions at school.

My son does occasionally "cheat" on his diet, and we still have an "accident" now and then (as ingredients in our favorite products change), but he is growing and remains relatively healthy. He is knowledgeable about his diet and realizes how sick he gets and miserable he feels when he eats gluten-containing foods. Although that knowledge has not ensured that he always makes the right food choices (his OCD and autism are factors in this rebellion), he is doing so much better. We are very grateful for the improvements we've seen since his "just for giggles" diagnosis.

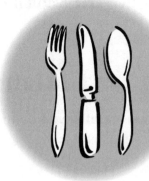

Chapter 1

A Guide to Gluten-Free Beginnings

"You tell me and I forget.
You teach me and I remember.
You involve me and I learn."
—Ben Franklin

As a parent, you do the best you can to protect your children from the woes of life: scraped knees, bee stings, broken hearts. You hope and pray that the pains your children do experience will teach them important life lessons like: don't run in the house, don't hit beehives with sticks, and be careful whom you trust. When you are trying to keep a child with gluten sensitivities healthy, caring for him takes a bit more preparation. Although keeping him on a special diet may seem like an overwhelming task at first, it does become more manageable with practice.

The key to the gluten-free diet is to identify and avoid foods that contain *gluten*—the insoluble protein component of wheat, rye, barley, and other grains. Since "gluten" is rarely listed as an ingredient in products that contain gluten, this chapter will cover the basics you need to know to identify gluten-containing foods and keep them from creeping into your child's diet.

Foods Allowed on the Gluten-Free Diet

The following grains/starches are **allowed** on the gluten-free diet:
- rice flour,
- potato flour,
- tapioca flour,
- bean flour,
- sorghum flour,
- soy flour,
- nut flours, and
- arrowroot.

Amaranth, buckwheat, millet, quinoa, and teff flours can be used but are *not* supported by all U.S. celiac disease support groups.

In addition, fresh fruits, vegetables, and meats are almost always gluten-free (some meats are minimally processed, so check the labels.) Many canned and frozen fruits, vegetables, and unprocessed meats are always gluten-free, as well as many dried products (e.g., canned tuna and pumpkin, frozen berries, frozen corn on the cob, sun-dried raisins, etc.).

Foods Not Allowed on the Gluten-Free Diet

The following grains contain gluten and are **not allowed:**
- wheat,
- rye,
- barley,
- spelt,
- triticale, and
- kamut.

Items that are listed as "wheat-free" do not necessarily mean gluten-free. Wheat-free products may still contain rye, barley, or other ingredients that are not gluten-free.

Questionable Foods

The following ingredients are **questionable** and **should not** be consumed unless you can verify that they do not contain or are not derived from prohibited grains:
- brown rice syrup (frequently made with barley),
- caramel color,

- dextrin (usually corn, but could be derived from wheat),
- flour or cereal products,
- hydrolyzed vegetable protein (HVP), vegetable protein, hydrolyzed plant protein (HPP), or textured vegetable protein (TVP),
- malt or malt flavoring (usually made from barley; okay if made from corn),
- modified food starch or modified starch (in the U.S., "food starch" is always corn starch),
- mono- & di-glycerides (in dry products only),
- natural flavors/artificial flavors,
- soy sauce or soy sauce solids (most soy sauces contain wheat),
- vegetable gum (made from oats),
- oats (chemically contains no gluten, yet has a high risk of cross contamination in the field due to crop rotations).

The following are additional components in processed foods that are frequently overlooked, and often contain gluten:
- breading,
- broth,
- coating mixes,
- croutons,
- imitation bacon,
- imitation seafood,
- marinades,
- pasta,
- roux,
- sauces,
- self-basting poultry,
- soup base,
- stuffing,
- thickeners.

Learn The Red Flags

This chapter provides a quick and simplistic view of the gluten-free diet. Not all areas of the diet are as clear-cut as portrayed in this chapter. These guidelines are intended as a safe, yet **temporary** survival tool until you can order and read a diet instruction manual, like the *Gluten Intolerance Group of North America's Gluten-Free Diet Instruction.* (See "Organizations and Support Groups" on page 311 in the Resources section for address and phone number for the Gluten Intolerance Group of North America.) With the assistance of a diet instruction manual, you will be able to read labels of food products, then determine if a product is gluten-free, not gluten-free, or questionable. Questionable ingredients do not give enough information to determine if it is gluten-free or not. An example of this is: modified food starch (the type of starch needs to be identified).

Finding a "clear" label is the safest way to find gluten-free food. A "clear" label is one that has no gluten-containing ingredients or questionable ingredients. If a food product you wish to eat has questionable ingredients, it is easier and safer to keep looking and try a comparable product with a clear label. You may clear the questionable ingredients by calling or writing to the food manufacturer, but some manufacturers change ingredients seasonally as prices or availability of foods change. For example, the malt flavoring that is clear today as being made from corn may change at any time to barley. Some foods remain gluten-free for years; others do not. Sometimes you get different information from the manufacturer each time you call. How you phrase questions (be positive and pleasant) and to whom you speak is important. It is best to talk to the food chemist or nutritionist, but it is often difficult to get past the public relations person. You'll need to be patient but diligent. **Remember, you must read the labels every time you purchase food.**

Involve your child in food selections and in the cooking process as soon as he or she is ready. Select some of the recipes that are designated as EASY so your child can learn about the gluten-free diet first hand. You need to allow your child to take ownership of his or her diet. You won't always be able to watch their every move. "Give your children the coping skills to deal with anything. Let them know it's okay to make a decision, then they'll do well with their challenges," said Mary Schluckebier, President of the Celiac Sprue Association of the United States of America (CSA/USA). Teach your child how to read labels as young as possible. Consider teaching your child the motto, "If in doubt, leave it out." Then be sure to share your knowledge with caregivers about your child's diet.

When you are adding a new food to your child's diet, particularly one that has questionable ingredients, introduce only one new food at a time. Wait a few days before adding any other new foods allowing time for a reaction, if any, to be linked to the new food that was added.

If In Doubt, Leave It Out

*If you are unable to clear the ingredients or the ingredients list is unavailable—***DO NOT ALLOW YOUR CHILD TO EAT IT!*** It is not worth triggering your child's immune system and/or damaging the small intestine. Every time a child with Celiac Disease consumes gluten, regardless of the amount, damage is done to the small intestine, even when the symptoms are not present.*

Organizing Your Kitchen:

Gluten-free foods being prepared must not come into contact with food containing gluten in any manner. Contamination may come from foods touching each other, being prepared on common surfaces, or with the utensils that are not thoroughly cleaned after preparing gluten-containing foods. For instance, flour sifters used for gluten-free ingredients should not be shared with gluten-containing flours. Deep frying gluten-free foods in oil used to fry gluten-containing products will contaminate them and should not be eaten.

To do the best job possible of keeping your kitchen safe from cross-contamination, you need to take some time to organize it. Look carefully at food storage, both the pantry and cold foods. Identify and organize an area for food preparation, food products, and cooking utensils. You want to be confident with food preparation, including helpful tips for in the kitchen and involving your child in food choices. Being consistent and calm will benefit you the most in the kitchen when you are preparing both gluten-free and gluten-containing foods.

Begin the process of organizing your kitchen with food storage. Start by thinking of how you can mark your gluten-free foods and designate safe areas of your kitchen. Then take a day to make your initial clean sweep through your kitchen. Remove food items from the cupboards and pantry to the floor or a box. Thoroughly clean each shelf and replace the shelf paper (if used). Planning and organizing your kitchen will make it easier for you (as well as anyone else who cares for your child in your home) to select safe foods for your child.

Where in your kitchen do you want to prepare your gluten-free foods? If possible, use the shelves that are closest to this designated preparation area to store gluten-free dry foods. When storing dry foods in containers, keep in mind that square and rectangular containers fit better on a shelf than do round ones. Label the contents of each container (if needed) and be consistent in keeping your gluten-free foods separate from your gluten-containing foods. Once you have identified foods as gluten-free, consider putting stickers (colored dots, stars, or mailing labels with "Gluten Free" printed on them from your computer, etc.) on the foods your child can have. Put these items in the area you have prepared for them.

Place the other foods in two piles, "contains gluten" and "questionable." You can confirm the ingredients in the questionable pile later, labeling and storing accordingly. Put the "contains gluten" foods on the shelves near the area designated for foods that contain gluten.

Now that you have organized your cupboards and pantry, you can do the same for cold storage in the refrigerator and freezer. Mark the packaging of freezer items with a freezer pen to reduce fading or smearing. Try to keep your gluten-free foods to one side or the other of the freezer and refrigerator. This practice may help prevent cross-contamination, but more likely will aid you in finding the foods you need more quickly.

For food preparation, think about items you should have duplicates of in order to prevent cross-contamination. Store the gluten-free dedicated kitchen utensils separately in the gluten-free part of your kitchen. Listed below are some items to think about duplicating.

Measuring tools:
- Set of measuring spoons
- Set of dry measuring cups
- Clear glass liquid measuring cups, 1 and 2 cup capacity

Mixing tools:
- Mixing bowls
- Colander
- Wooden or acrylic spoons
- Rubber spatula
- Flour sifter
- Flexible metal spatula (great for leveling dry ingredients)
- Wire whisk (whip)
- Pancake turners
- Metal tongs

Cutting tools:
- Paring knife
- Serrated bread knife
- Kitchen shears
- Cutting board
- Food chopper
- Grater and/or shredder

Bakeware:
- Wire cooling rack
- Rolling pin
- Pastry brushes, ½ inch to 2 inches
- Cake pans—round, square, or rectangular
- Bread machine pan
- Loaf pan—for bread, meat loaves, etc.
- Muffin pan—6 or 12 muffin cups
- Pastry wheel
- Pastry blender
- Pizza pan or stone
- Cookie press
- Cookie sheet(s)

Food Preparation

Many people like to use a bread machine to prepare both their gluten-free and gluten-containing breads. The two schools of thought are 1) to have a dedicated bread machine for your gluten-free bread baking or 2) to purchase a replacement bread pan and mark it "Gluten-Free Only." The first option is the safest, if you can afford and/or store two bread machines. The second option works as long as you are careful to clean your bread machine in between batches of bread, like the lid and surfaces that the bread can touch outside of the bread pan. Separate bread pans are needed because the paddles sit on a rubberized seal that is somewhat porous. The seal can contain miniscule particles of gluten. The gluten particles on the seal and on the paddle are next to impossible to remove completely. Therefore, if you use a single bread machine to prepare your gluten-free and gluten-containing breads, have a dedicated bread pan just for the gluten-free bread.

Using a common toaster for gluten-free bread and regular bread is a major source of contamination. Consider toasting your gluten-free bread in a separate, dedicated toaster or on separate, dedicated racks in the toaster oven. Clean the toaster or toaster oven often to remove accumulated crumbs. If a second toaster is not feasible, consider pan toast (see page 96). You just might throw that old toaster out after all!

When you begin to prepare food, such as a sandwich or toast, start by placing your bread (either gluten-free or not) on a plate or paper towel. Use separate knives for gluten-containing and gluten-free breads. To spread jam, etc. on your sandwich, use a spoon to take the product from the jar. Do not wipe the excess jam on the knife from spreading back into the jar; the jam is now full of crumbs. Even the most discerning eye won't be able to tell gluten-free crumbs from gluten-containing crumbs in a jar of jam. Other options, if you have the storage space:

1. have a dedicated, gluten-free jar of jam, mayonnaise, peanut butter, etc. or
2. put these products in squeeze bottles for everyone to use.

The butter dish is an especially "crummy" place. You may wish to follow Miss Manners' advice and place butter on the table with its own butter knife, which touches no food excepting the butter. The butter is placed on your plate with the communal knife; then with your own butter knife, spread on whatever you choose to put your butter on. It does effectively keep the crumbs out of the butter as well as returning to some good, old-fashioned manners.

What about those quick, hot meals? Even zapping leftovers in the microwave for a few seconds will require more planning. Use clean microwave dishes or paper towels under <u>all</u> foods you heat in the microwave to prevent contaminating your gluten-free foods. Clean your microwave often, especially if an item has "splattered" the inside of your microwave. This will assist in preventing not only gluten-contamination, but also germs and bacteria that grow on the "splattered" food. After all, you are doing the best that you can to keep your family healthy.

Reducing Stress in Food Preparation

Now for some advice to keep your gluten-free kitchen filled with reduced-stress dressing on a crispy bed of contentment.

First, get into the habit of cleaning up as you work: it helps in the preparation process, cuts down the risk of cross-contamination, and reduces the risk of mistakes.

Second, consider setting out all the ingredients before starting a recipe, then put the items away as they are used. After all, you are cooking for your child, so this plan may help you to keep up with where you left off should (or when) you get interrupted. (Beware of little hands trying to help you by putting their yogurt-covered raisins in the bread dough while you answer the phone.)

Third, consider using colored plastic wrap (like pink—to symbolize caution) on the leftover foods such as spaghetti that contain gluten but are not as easily recognizable in the refrigerator.

Fourth, be creative! Mary Schluckebier, of CSA/USA, suggests having a family meeting to ask these questions:

1. "What foods would you wish we never ran out of?"
2. "What foods would you wish we never ate again?"

Try to work in more foods from the first question and less foods from the second question. What if your child doesn't like vegetables? Be creative and offer your child some solutions. (I have been known to add finely shredded carrots to, say … pizza crust, or spinach leaves to lasagna! However, I do occasionally get caught.)

Fifth, to manage your grocery budget more effectively, consider buying your products in bulk. Store your bulk items in large, plastic containers. Store your large containers in the floor of a closet or in your garage. Buying in bulk reduces your cost and helps with that stressful feeling of "Oh no! I'm out of gluten-free pasta! Now how do I put together this creative spinach lasagna without the pasta?" To be productive in the kitchen with less stress, simply follow this advice and smile often.

There is one last important decision to make if you have a child on a gluten-free diet:

1. should the whole family eat gluten-free meals,
2. should the whole family eat reduced gluten-meals, or
3. should just your child eat gluten-free meals?

This is a personal decision that has many aspects to ponder. Is the cost a factor? Do you have the time to prepare two dishes for each meal? This decision may require some thought, research, trial, and error to discover what works best for your family.

The recipes in this book taste good enough for your entire family to eat them. The proportions in the book are designed for the entire family. You may want to change the proportions of the recipes or be prepared to freeze some portions to use later if you are preparing gluten-free foods for just the child on the gluten-free diet.

In this day and age, most parents hardly have time to prepare one meal, so preparing two meals seems like an enormous task. If your entire family is not on the gluten-free diet, paying attention to food preparation habits, being organized, and *doing the best that you can* will eliminate most of your concerns of cross-contamination in your home. Remember that changing to a gluten-free diet is more of a lifestyle change than a simple diet change.

*(Some information in this section was adapted from the **Gluten Intolerance Group of North America's** "Quick Start Guide," used with permission.)*

Chapter 2

Understanding Celiac Disease

Some children may begin a gluten-free diet because they have a food allergy. Other children may begin a gluten-free (and perhaps also dairy-free diet, as a way to manage autism. However, a large number of children will begin a gluten-free diet as the result of a diagnosis of celiac disease.

This cookbook is not exclusively for families who have children with celiac disease, but a large percentage of users of this book will likely fall into that category. The following information is meant to provide a brief understanding of celiac disease and the issues associated with it for parents who are new to the diagnosis, or perhaps only suspect that their child may have celiac disease.

What Is Celiac Disease?

The word "celiac" is derived from the Greek word "koiliakos," which means "suffering in the bowels." We now know that this suffering is caused by a sensitivity to gluten in food that results in inflammation and atrophy (wasting away) of the lining of the small intestine. Over time, repeated exposure to gluten damages the *villi* in the intestinal lining—small hair-like projections that ordinarily absorb nutrients from digested food. A variety of symptoms can appear once the small intestine has been damaged, including chronic diarrhea, malnutrition, bloating, and other symptoms discussed below. Celiac disease is not an allergy, but an autoimmune disorder—a condition in which the body produces immune reactions against itself, leading to tissue damage.

Celiac disease is found most often in countries where wheat is a staple food. It is especially common in European countries such as Ireland, Italy, Sweden, Germany, and Finland, or in places such as Australia or North America, where there are many people of European descent. Few cases of celiac disease are diagnosed in African and Asian countries. However, when people from Africa or Asia immigrate into societies consuming gluten, these populations show surprising rates of celiac disease. Therefore, the reduced occurrence of celiac disease in African and Asian countries may be more from little-to-no gluten consumption, lower genetic susceptibility, or simply a lack of proper diagnosis.

In the United States, studies are being conducted to discover just how many people have celiac disease. Current statistics from a study by Dr. Alessio Fasano at the University of Maryland show that one in 250 adults and one in 400 children in the United States have celiac disease. (Compare this to the rate of diabetes of one in 500 people.) These statistics do not include the many adults and children with simple food allergies to wheat, rye, and/or barley (WRB).

Symptoms of Celiac Disease

The symptoms of celiac disease vary widely with the age of the patient, length of exposure to gluten, and level of the disease before being diagnosed. Celiac disease can be compared to an iceberg. The tip of the iceberg, the part that is easy to recognize, consists of the classic or typical symptoms. Beneath the surface, there may also be atypical (uncharacteristic) and latent (hidden) symptoms. Classic (typical) symptoms include:

- chronic diarrhea,
- failure to thrive,
- a big, bloated (or distended) tummy.

The atypical (uncharacteristic) symptoms can include:

- dermatitis herpetiformis (an itchy, blistering skin rash),
- short stature,
- tooth enamel deficiencies,
- iron-deficient anemia,
- arthritis and joint pain,
- osteoporosis,
- neurological problems or diseases,
- delays in onset of puberty,
- infertility,
- increased risk of miscarriages,
- chronic hepatitis and liver damage.

Silent (latent) symptoms include:
- iron-deficiency, with or without anemia,
- weakened physical fitness (often tired and easily fatigued),
- decline in behavioral health (irritability, depression, impaired performance at school with children),
- lowered bone mineral mass.

In addition, there are many disorders that are associated with an increased risk of celiac disease. People who have these disorders may be asymptomatic (show no symptoms) for celiac disease for much or all of their lives, but have an increased likelihood of developing it. Associated medical conditions/autoimmune disorders (asymptomatic) can include:
- thyroid disorders,
- hepatitis disorders,
- degeneratative stomach disorders,
- Addison disease,
- Sjogren syndrome,
- Down syndrome,
- Turner syndrome,
- Williams syndrome,
- IgA deficiency,
- hereditary heart defects.

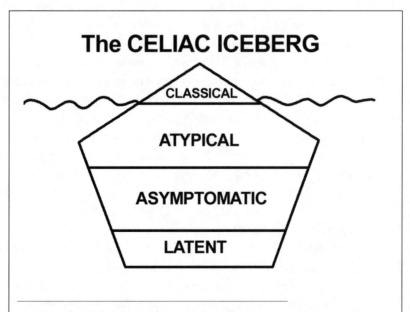

Courtesy of Dr. Karoly Horvath, Center for Celiac Research, University of Maryland Medical School (Horvath K. Celiac Disease. Recent Advances in Pediatrics-12. Jaypee Brothers, Medical Publishers Ltd., 2002, pp: 1-23). Used with permission.

Celiac Disease and Malnutrition

By Cynthia Kupper, RD, CD, Executive Director, Gluten Intolerance Group™

Until recently, malnutrition was the hallmark of celiac disease. (In children, symptoms of malnutrition include legs and arms that look like skin and bones and a bloated stomach.) That is changing, as people of all ages are being diagnosed before the severe stages of malnutrition occur. Yet malnutrition is still a concern. Often the initial signs of malnutrition are subtle–drier skin, dull hair, changes in fingernails, fatigue, memory problems, delayed puberty, short stature. Although you may not realize there is a problem, damage in the small intestine caused by untreated or undiagnosed celiac disease is a concern for all persons with celiac disease–especially children.

Digestion and absorption of food starts in the mouth with the production of saliva. The stomach acts as a mixer and blender, combining stomach secretions with the food to break it down into smaller pieces and mix it together well. From there, this chyme (or slurry of food and juices) moves into the small intestine. This is where the real work of digestion happens. From the beginning of the uppermost part of the small intestine, the chyme is broken down further and absorbed into the body as precursors of nutrients or nutrients themselves.

Celiac disease damage usually begins at the top of the small intestine and works its way down. Healing is thought to be the reverse process. Most vitamins, minerals, and nutrients—such as carbohydrates—are absorbed in the uppermost one-third of the small intestine—where the major part of the damage occurs in celiac disease. Thus, when children have damage to this part of their small intestine, they may have very low levels of certain nutrients, such as B vitamins, zinc, magnesium, and iron. Most of these nutrients are restored to normal levels with the healing of the small intestine and a simple multi-vitamin supplement. In the case of iron deficiencies, however, larger doses may be required for a period of time. Always consult your health care team before giving your child mega-doses of vitamins and minerals.

If the intestinal damage progresses beyond the upper part of the small intestine, your child may have additional symptoms. This is because protein, fat-soluble vitamins, and fats are absorbed in the middle to lower part of the small intestine. People who malabsorb fats have diarrhea and floating, frothy stools that are very odorous. If the diagnosis of celiac disease is made early, most people will not have damage in the lower part of the small intestine. This explains why all children with celiac disease do not have diarrhea or foul-smelling stools.

The Treatment: The Gluten-Free Diet

The gluten-free diet is the prescribed medical treatment for celiac disease, as well as for dermatitis herpetiformis (a blistering rash on the skin, usually around the knees, elbows, or buttocks, that some people get after consuming gluten.) Staying on a strict gluten-free diet usually leads to the complete healing of the lining of the small intestine. On the whole, the younger the patient starts the gluten-free diet, the more dramatic the improvement tends to be.

The gluten-free diet for the treatment of celiac disease is a *lifelong* commitment and should not be started unless your child is properly diagnosed. A biopsy showing damaged villi in the small intestine is the "gold standard" to being diagnosed with celiac disease. (See photos of villi below.) A skin biopsy confirms dermatitis herpetiformis. Starting the diet without complete testing is not recommended

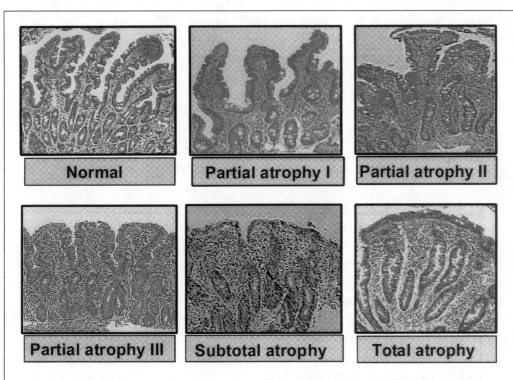

These photographs show how the consumption of gluten progressively damages the intestinal villi in individuals with celiac disease. The first photo is normal, healthy intestinal villi. The "Total atrophy" can be expected with classic symptoms of celiac disease. The variations in between these examples are also positive for celiac disease, but can be expected in atypical to latent forms of the disease

Courtesy of Dr. Karoly Horvath, Center for Celiac Research, University of Maryland Medical School (Horvath K. Celiac Disease. Recent Advances in Pediatrics-12. Jaypee Brothers, Medical Publishers Ltd., 2002, pp: 1-23). Used with permission.

because it makes diagnosis difficult. Tests to confirm celiac disease would be negative if a person were on the gluten-free diet for very long. A valid test would require reintroducing gluten (a gluten challenge) before testing.

Since celiac disease is an inherited autoimmune digestive disease, proper diagnosis of your child can be very important to other members of the family. A positive diagnosis will help relatives and future generations be aware of the risk of celiac disease within the family.

Not All Adverse Reactions Are Due to Celiac Disease

Lactose intolerance; food sensitivities or allergies to soy, corn, or other foods; or the stomach flu are common causes of similar symptoms to celiac disease. In addition, children who have been newly diagnosed with celiac disease may still have trouble tolerating certain foods, especially fatty foods, until the small intestine has had a chance to heal and start working normally. When attempting to determine why your child could be having diarrhea or other adverse reactions, read labels, remember what was eaten (or use the food intake record on pages 18-19), and listen to your child's body.

The History of Celiac Disease

Celiac disease was first written about in the second century A.D. by Aretaeus of Cappadocia, a contemporary of the ancient Roman physician, Galen. It was Aretaeus who coined the Greek word "koiliakos" to describe people with celiac disease. When that word passed through Latin to the modern English of the 1800s, it became "coeliac," which is how "celiac" is still spelled in Great Britain. (Both terms refer to the same disease.)

It wasn't until 1888 that the next clear clinical account of childhood and adult celiac conditions was given by Samuel Jones Gee, M.D., of London. For a time, the condition became known as Gee's Disease.

During the early part of the twentieth century, the doctors most accountable for increasing our knowledge of celiac disease were caring for pediatric patients. The first book on the celiac condition was published in 1908 by Dr. Christian Archibald Herter, of Connecticut. He became such an expert on the condition that it was often referred to as Gee-Herter's Disease. Herter's most important contribution was his statement that people with the condition tolerate fats better than carbohydrates. Sir Frederick Still, another pediatrician, first drew attention to the specific harmful effects of bread in 1918, stating, "Unfortunately one form of starch which seems particularly liable to aggravate the symptoms is bread. I know of no adequate substitute." In 1921, the American Pediatric Society was recommending that children with celiac disease be treated with a diet that rigorously excluded carbohydrates. Three years later, in 1924, came the banana diet, which was essentially a diet low in carbohydrates except for ripe bananas.

The fundamental discovery in the treatment of children with celiac disease came after World War II. The discovery was made and described in detail by a Dutch pediatrician, Professor Willem Karel Dicke, in his doctoral thesis in 1950. He described how children with celiac disease had benefited dramatically during the war when wheat, oats, and rye flour were rationed. The children's appetites had returned, their absorption of fat had improved, and their diarrhea had disappeared. After the war, when the children resumed consuming wheat, oats, and rye flours, they became sick once more.

The next breakthrough in the understanding of celiac disease came when Dr. J. W. Paulley of Ipswich described to the British Society of Gastroenterology an inflammation of the lining of the small intestine in an adult celiac patient. This inflammation was then confirmed in several other patients with celiac disease. This discovery has become the most essential single feature on which the diagnosis of celiac disease is based.

In the past ten to fifteen years, the medical community has discovered that celiac disease is much more prevalent than originally thought. Many new forms of testing have been and are continuing to be developed to assist in the diagnosis of celiac disease. A worldwide research effort has been launched in an effort to understand more about the celiac condition. Future directions of research in celiac disease have been clearly defined at the 9th International Symposium on Celiac Disease in 2000 and at the first World Congress of Pediatric Gastroenterology, Hepatology, and Nutrition in the same year. The world of science has now begun to appreciate that celiac disease is not a condition confined to Europe, as was previously thought, but has global implications.

The Beginning

If your child has been diagnosed with celiac disease, there are many reasons to be optimistic. Celiac disease *can* be managed. There are no medications required. Children and adults with celiac disease recover fully and can expect to live normal, fulfilling lives if they faithfully follow the gluten-free diet. The diagnosis of celiac disease is not the end of the world for your child. On the contrary, it is the beginning of a healthy, happy life full of all the adventures, hopes, and desires of any other child.

Food Intake Record

Date started: _____   Day of week: _____

Record food intake for 3 to 5 days

Remember to:

- Record all meals, snacks, and fluids taken by your child.
- Include brand names.
- Indicate times of meals and snacks.
- Record food and fluid amounts in teaspoons, tablespoons, cups, ounces, etc.

DATE	TIME	FOOD OR DRINK	DESCRIPTION (how prepared or brand name)	AMOUNT EATEN
Example:				
3/23	7:00 AM	Orange Juice	From frozen concentrate	½ cup
"	"	Buttermilk Pancake	Recipe from *Incredible Edible* cookbook	1 4-inch whole
"	"	Butter	Lucerne	2 tsp.
"	"	Maple Syrup	Mrs. Butterworth's Lite	2 Tbsp.
"	"	Milk	Whole	1 cup

DATE	TIME	FOOD OR DRINK	DESCRIPTION (how prepared or brand name)	AMOUNT EATEN

This chart will help you keep up with your child's calorie intake, relieve your mind that your child really is eating, and give you information to take to your doctor or dietitian. Children often consume *less* food than before going on the gluten-free diet, simply because they are now absorbing the nutrients in the food.

(This chart may be photocopied as needed for personal use only.)

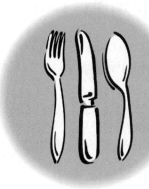

Chapter 3

Special Help for Your Child

"Feelings are real and legitimate;
children behave and misbehave for a reason,
even if adults cannot figure it out."
—*Unknown*

There are many reasons for you and your child to resist changing his (or her) lifestyle to the gluten-free diet. It is not easy, at first, to identify and remove all the gluten from the diet. Children get very attached to their favorite foods (as do we, the parents). How can your child ever *live* without pizza, sandwiches, doughnuts, or whatever favorite food you or your child thinks must be a part of a happy childhood?

Emotions aside, there are many reasons for children with celiac disease to stay on the gluten-free diet. Some, but probably not all, of these reasons usually apply to children with a gluten intolerance or allergy as well. They include:

- to regain health,
- to be able to grow (again),
- to reduce and eliminate symptoms such as tummy aches, anemia, diarrhea, constipation, headaches, and itchy rashes, to name a few,
- to reduce susceptibility to other illnesses, such as the common cold, bone loss, and vitamin deficiencies, and possibly reduce the likelihood of juvenile diabetes, neurological disorders, and cancers,

- to be able to focus on having a childhood, not an illness,
- to feel GOOD!

There are also many downsides to continuing on a "typical" diet for children with celiac disease. (Again, some, but not all of these may apply to children with a gluten intolerance or allergy.)

- costly medical procedures,
- school absences (resulting in more homework and less play time),
- emotional disturbances (such as depression),
- perhaps, even a shorter lifespan due to malnutrition (caused by celiac disease).

Clearly, it is to your child's advantage to stay on the gluten-free diet for life if he or she is diagnosed with celiac disease. There are also many advantages for children with a gluten intolerance or allergy, although they may or may not need to stay on the diet all their lives. How you teach your child to cope will help tremendously when that temptation does come up.

Coping with Food Temptations

What can you teach your child to say when someone offers her a gluten-containing item? First, your child will need to decide whether the offer is made out of kindness (willingness to share) or just to be mean (peer pressure.)

When someone merely wants to share, the best, simplest approach is for your child to be honest. She can reply with a comment such as: "No, thank you. I have a medically required diet, but thank you anyway." Any caring person will accept this kind of approach and usually be very helpful in the future concerning your child's diet.

If someone is tempting your child to be mean or unkind, you will need to teach your child to defend herself with a positive attitude toward herself and her diet. One approach most kids can relate to is "The Poison Ivy Approach." Teach your child to ask her tormentor, "Would you sit in a huge patch of poison ivy on purpose?" (Of course not.) "So why would I eat foods I am not supposed to when I know how sick I will get if I eat them?" No treat is worth that miserable feeling. Another approach, "The Anti-Peer Pressure Approach," can be used for the bullies your child may encounter. "Would you jump out in front of a speeding truck, even if I tell you it won't hurt you that bad?" ("Well, uh, no.") "Then why are you pressuring me to eat something that is really bad for me, even if it is okay for you?"

Your child will need to learn to be her own best friend when it comes to managing her food. Help her gain the tools necessary to be self-confident, self-disciplined, and self-controlled.

If your child has speech delays due to autism, Down syndrome, etc., you can have your child wear a button or carry a note that says something like "I have a medically required diet. Please do not offer me foods. Ask my (mom, dad, caregiver, etc.) to check that the food you want to share is okay for my diet. Thank you."

Childcare and School

Letting your child go out into the world by herself can be stressful for any parent in today's busy society. Your concerns can be magnified when your child needs to follow a special diet, particularly when she is not old enough to advocate for herself. Making sure that adults in your child's environment are aware of dietary concerns are often especially big issues at daycare and school. Here are some hints to ensuring that your child's special needs will be taken care of appropriately while in a daycare or school setting.

Daycare Issues

When selecting a daycare or child care for your young child with celiac disease or gluten intolerance, interview the staff carefully. If your child is already enrolled in a daycare center or receiving care in someone else's home when she begins the gluten-free diet, you will also need to educate the staff about your child's new needs. Here are some things to pay particular attention to.

- **Make sure food facilities are clean:** Where do children eat? Where is food prepared? Are children constantly supervised during meals so that stray crumbs don't end up on your child's plate?
- **Coordinate snacks:** If the provider lists a menu ahead of time you may be able to provide similar gluten-free snacks for your child.
- **Coordinate birthday celebrations:** Store frozen frosted mini-cakes at home or at the daycare. Your child can participate with a gluten-free cake that has been defrosted.
- **Coordinate lunches:** Be sure the food provided is gluten-free or provide your child's lunch.
- **Coordinate tactile play:** Be sure that the craft items your child will be playing with are gluten-free or provide a gluten-free alternative. Specific items to look for are play dough, silly putty, finger paints, and stringing items such as cereal O's or noodles. (See pages 267-273 for gluten-free craft recipes.)
- **Consider a medical alert bracelet, anklet, or button:** Even a "Don't Feed Me Wheat" button with a cute picture can be a constant reminder to your child's care provider.

- **Inform the staff about reactions:** Connect with the director, teacher, or provider to inform them about how your child reacts to gluten, as well as the absolute necessity to follow your directions.

Remember, if the daycare/child care provider won't work with you, find someone else who will. Your child's health depends on it.

Preschool Issues

Plan to interview staff at preschools as you did for the daycare/child care providers, especially if your child is still quite young or has some communication difficulties. Here are some additional things to pay particular attention to.

- **Communicate with your child:** Explain to your child why some crafts or games are *not* okay for him. Continue to make sure that the craft items your child will be playing with are gluten-free. Politely offer to provide the gluten-free alternative.
- **Teach your child to ask about ingredients:** You need to be sure the food or snacks are gluten-free or provide your child's food, but encourage your child to take ownership of her own diet.
- **Provide a reminder:** Remember to discuss your child's food intolerances with your child's care providers.
- **Inform the preschool about reactions:** Inform the director, teacher, and/or provider about how your child reacts to gluten, as well as the need to follow your directions concerning food consumption.
- **Encourage your child's feedback:** Encourage your child to express her feelings or frustrations about her food intolerance, allergy, or celiac condition in words or pictures. Share the pictures with others to help them understand how your child feels.

Again, if the preschool won't work with you, find one that will.

Elementary School and Beyond

- **Make communication a major goal in your child's life:** Encourage your child to share his feelings and frustrations with you in a respectful manner.
- **Discourage your child from "trading" lunches:** If necessary, talk to cafeteria staff or lunchroom aides about your child's need to avoid gluten-containing foods.
- **Talk with your child's teacher often.**
- **Continue to coordinate**: Plan and coordinate crafts, birthday celebrations, and lunch concerns with the school.

Community Activities

As your child gets older, more and more activities will be a part of her life. Keep your lines of communication open and respectful. As your child's lifestyle becomes busier, remember the tips above and continue to:

- Inform,
- Teach,
- Supply.

Pay particular attention to the information needs of anyone who may plan activities for your child that require food or access to food, including parents of friends, grandparents, aunts, uncles, church leaders, Sunday school teachers, Girl/Boy Scout leaders, 4-H club leaders, sports coaches, dance instructors, camp directors, and counselors.

Show Your Child the Way

You know your child better than anyone else does. It is important that you be her advocate. Help your child adjust to the lifestyle change of the gluten-free diet. Keep the lines of communication open with your child, her childcare providers, school teachers, activity leaders, and especially her physician.

Teach your child how to cook and bake. As soon as your child is ready, have her help you in the kitchen. Soon your child will be enjoying her gluten-free lifestyle as much as the one she left behind, plus she will be well enough to really enjoy her childhood.

Chapter 4

Before You Start

"It's always too soon to quit."
—Anon.

Before you prepare a recipe for the first time, read it through carefully to be sure that you have everything you will need. Avoid doubling or halving a recipe the first time: sometimes it can be done successfully, but not always. It's always a good idea to follow the recipe exactly, within your dietary limits, the first time. If substitutions *are required*, for optimal results use the substitutions suggested in **Cooking Tips** at the back of the book.

Do as much preparation in advance before you start mixing and/or cooking a recipe. Be careful to measure and mix accurately. Advance preparation of your equipment is also important. Greasing pans and preheating the oven are most often the steps that save you time in your food preparation, and possibly even save your recipe.

Get into the habit of cleaning up as you work: it helps in the preparation process, cuts down the risk of cross-contamination in the kitchen (if you still use any gluten-containing foods), and reduces the risk of mistakes.

You'll want to involve your child in the cooking process as soon as she is ready. It gives your child ownership of her diet, as well as reducing the desire to "cheat." Some recipes have been marked "EASY" (E*z*) so you can select some for a younger child to cook with you. Recipes that are marked with a "clock" ( ) can be prepared quickly, in under 30 minutes. Recipes that are marked with a "hand" (🖐) are finger foods. In the Index, you can find separate lists of EASY, FAST, or Finger Foods.

Common Ingredients

Most of the ingredients called for in these recipes can be found in any grocery store. If you have an allergy to some of them, check out page 276 for substitutions. Here is a list of common ingredients found in this book.

- Corn starch
- Corn meal
- Unflavored gelatin
- Sugar
- Brown sugar
- Honey
- Molasses
- Powdered sugar
- Corn syrup, light
- Maple syrup
- Vegetable oil
- Olive oil
- Shortening
- Margarine
- Butter
- Baking powder
- Baking soda
- Active dry yeast
- Milk (or milk substitute)
- Dry milk
- Whipping cream
- Sour cream
- Yogurt
- Evaporated milk
- Egg replacer

- Eggs
- Salt
- Pepper
- Spices
- Herbs
- Vanilla
- Mayonnaise
- Prepared mustard
- Rice vinegar
- Apple cider vinegar
- Ketchup
- Worcestershire sauce
- Steak sauce
- Gluten-free soy sauce (such as Tamari™ or Braggs Amino Acids™)
- Bouillon granules, chicken & beef
- Meats
- Poultry
- Fish
- Cheeses
- Salad greens
- Vegetables
- Fruit juices
- Fruits
- Nuts

Specialty Ingredients

Some recipes call for ingredients that you may never have used before, or that are difficult to find in many grocery stores. These ingredients can be ordered from the Gluten-Free Suppliers listed at the back of the book if you can't find them locally. Specialty ingredients used in these recipes include:

- Rice flour—a finely ground flour made from white rice.
- Brown rice flour—a finely ground flour made from brown rice. More nutritious than rice flour, it has a nutty flavor and is a good source of fiber.
- Sweet rice flour—a finely ground flour made from a short-grained white rice, good for thickening and baking. Sometimes found in the Chinese section of larger grocery stores.
- Tapioca flour—a very fine powder made from the leaves of the Cassava plant. Adds "chew" to a recipe. (Not the same as tapioca for pudding available at grocery stores.)
- Potato starch flour—a very fine powder, made from white potatoes. Absorbs moisture in a recipe. (Not the same as potato flour.)
- Potato flour—a fine powder, slightly yellow, with a strong potato flavor.
- Garfava flour—a fine powdered flour, made from a mix of garbanzo beans and fava beans, with a distinct flavor. High in protein and fiber.
- Xanthan gum—a very fine powder that provides elasticity in baked goods made without gluten. (Do not get wet during cleanup.)
- Buttermilk powder—a fine powdered milk product, used for baking, available through Ener-G Foods and other gluten-free suppliers.
- Gluten-free pastas—a basic staple food, many varieties and shapes are available, usually made from corn, rice, or quinoa & corn. (**See Gluten-Free Suppliers**, pages 295-300.)

Enjoy cooking and eating with your **Incredible Edible Gluten-Free Food for Kids** cookbook as your guide!

Appetizers & Snacks

Breads

Breakfast Ideas

RECIPES

Lunch & Dinner Ideas

Salads & Vegetables

Soups & Stews

Sweet Treats

Party & Entertaining Tips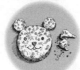

Just for Fun

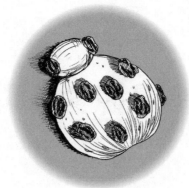

Appetizers & Snacks

"If your children look up to you, you've made a success of life's biggest job."

—Unknown

Baked Potato Skins

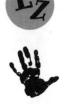

Ingredients

3 medium baking potatoes
2 tablespoons margarine or butter
½-1 cup shredded cheddar or Monterey Jack cheese (2-4 ounces)

Directions
Preheat oven to 425 degrees.

1. Wash potatoes and scrub well. Prick several times with a fork.
2. Place potatoes on center rack of 425-degree oven and bake for 40-50 minutes or until tender. Remove from oven.
3. Cut the baked potatoes in half, lengthwise, and scoop out the insides, leaving ½-inch thick shells.(Reserve pulp for another use.)
4. Brush the potato shells inside and out with melted margarine.
5. Place on an ungreased baking sheet with the cut side up.
6. Bake for 10-15 minutes or until crispy.
7. Fill loosely with the cheese.
8. Bake an additional 2-3 minutes or until the cheese is melted.
9. Serve with sour cream, bacon bits, and chives, if desired.

Makes 6 servings.

Buggy Bananas

Sometimes it is fun to play with your food.

Ingredients

2 tablespoons sweetened flaked coconut
1-2 drops food color of choice (optional)
1 banana
2 raisins
¼-½ teaspoon peanut butter, or other nut butter of choice.
Almond slivers

Directions

1. In a cereal-sized bowl, combine the flaked coconut with the food color, if used. Stir until the coconut has absorbed the food color and is evenly tinted.
2. Slice the banana into ¼ inch pieces.
3. Dip the top of each banana slice into the coconut mixture. On a plate, arrange the coated banana slices, coconut side up, in a swirling pattern. (See illustration.)
4. Dip a raisin into the peanut butter. "Glue" the raisin "eye" to one side of the first coated banana slice. Repeat with the other raisin.
5. Cut or break almond slivers in half. Dip one half of a sliver into the peanut butter and "glue" on an "antenna" behind the "eye" on the first banana slice. Repeat with the other "antenna." Dip the remaining sliver halves in the peanut butter and glue on as "legs" on each side of the remaining banana slices.

Makes one serving.

Brown Rice Crackers

Ingredients

- 1 cup brown rice flour
- 3 tablespoons gluten-free soy sauce
- ½ teaspoon sesame seeds
- 10 tablespoons of water

Directions
Preheat oven to 300 degrees.

1. In a small bowl, combine rice flour and sesame seeds.
2. In a separate small bowl, combine soy sauce and water. Add to the flour mixture and combine until smooth.
3. Drop mixture by measuring tablespoons onto a lightly oiled cookie sheet. Flatten with the bottom of a glass slightly oiled and dipped in brown rice flour, or flatten with fingers.
4. Bake in 300-degree oven for 40-45 minutes.

Makes about 20 crackers.
Store cooled crackers in a zip-style bag for up to two weeks.

Cheesy Tortillas

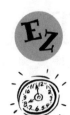

Ingredients

6 Corn Tortillas (or Rice Flour Tortillas)
1½ cups shredded cheddar or Monterey Jack Cheese

Directions

Preheat oven to 425 degrees.

1. Wrap the tortillas in foil and heat in a 425-degree oven for 10 minutes to soften.
2. Fill each tortilla with ¼ cup of shredded cheese and wrap, burrito-style, and place on an ungreased baking sheet.
3. Bake in 425-degree oven for 10 minutes or until cheese is melted.

Microwave Directions

1. Place the tortillas in a stack on a microwavable plate. Slightly moisten a paper (or linen) towel with water. Cover the tortillas with the moistened towel.
2. Heat the tortillas on high for about one minute to soften.
3. Fill each tortilla with ¼ cup shredded cheese and wrap, burrito-style, and place on a microwavable plate.
4. Heat the tortillas on high for about one minute or until the cheese is melted.

Makes 3 servings.

Deviled Eggs

Ingredients

> 6 hard-boiled eggs, cooled and peeled
> ¼ cup mayonnaise or salad dressing
> 1 teaspoon sugar
> 1 teaspoon apple vinegar
> 1 teaspoon prepared mustard
> 1 teaspoon sweet relish (optional)
> Ground paprika (optional)

Directions

1. Slice eggs in half lengthwise and carefully press egg yolks into a small bowl. Arrange the egg white halves on a plate or serving dish.
2. Mash the egg yolks with a fork or electric hand mixer on low. Add the mayonnaise, sugar, vinegar, mustard, and relish, if used. Blend well until smooth.
3. Spoon mixture into egg white halves using two spoons. (Use the second spoon to remove the egg yolk mixture from the first spoon.) Sprinkle with paprika for color and garnish, if desired.

Makes 1 dozen deviled eggs.

Variation: Instead of spooning the filling into the egg white halves, load filling into a cake-decorating bag with a large star tip. Pipe the egg yolk filling into the egg white halves and then sprinkle with the paprika. Garnish with a sprig or two of fresh parsley, if desired.

Juicy Kool-Aid®

To prepare a Kool-Aid® drink without any refined sugar, try this recipe. It's a hit with parents and their kids!

Ingredients

1 package unsweetened Kool Aid® powder, any flavor
½ gallon apple or white grape juice

Directions

1. Add the Kool-Aid® powder directly to the juice.
2. Shake or stir well and serve chilled or over ice.

Ladybugs

This is a fun snack that you and your child can make together.

Ingredients

1 medium-sized red apple
Raisins
Peanut butter or other nut butter
2 grapes (or whole almonds)

Directions

1. Wash the apple and cut in half. Remove the stem, blossom, and seeds.
2. Place each apple half on a small plate, cut side down.
3. Dip raisins in the peanut butter and use as "glue" to attach the raisins to the apple.
4. Dip one end of a grape in the peanut butter and attach to the stem side of the apple.
5. Dip two raisins in the peanut butter, and "glue" to the grape for eyes.

Makes 2 ladybugs. Enjoy eating your snack as much as you did making it!

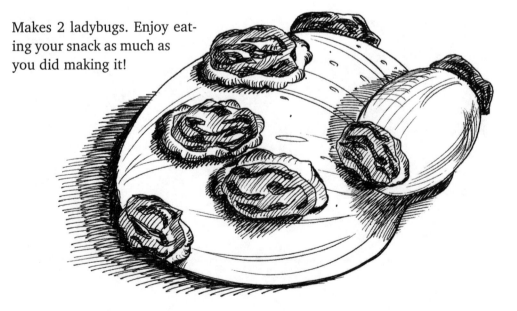

Nachos

Ingredients

> 4 cups corn tortilla chips or potato chips
> 1½ cups shredded cheddar cheese
> Toppings of choice, see below

Directions

Preheat oven to 350 degrees.

1. Arrange chips on a cookie sheet.
2. Top with shredded cheddar cheese and toppings, if desired.
3. Heat in 350-degree oven for 5-7 minutes or until the cheese is melted.

Makes 4 one-cup servings.

Toppings

> ½ cup shredded cooked chicken, turkey, or beef
> ½ cup sliced black olives
> ½ cup chopped green onions
> 1 4-ounce can diced green chilies, drained
> 1 cup cooked ground turkey or beef
> ½ cup gluten-free refried beans

Peanut-Free Trail Mix

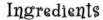

Ingredients

½ cup raw cashews (2½ ounces)
1 cup almond slices (5 ounces)
1 cup walnut pieces (5 ounces)
½ cup pecan pieces (2 ounces)
½ cup dates (4 ounces)*
2 tablespoons honey
2 tablespoons rice bran
1 cup golden raisins (2½-3 ounces)
1 cup raisins (2½-3 ounces)
¾ cup shredded, sweetened coconut (2 ounces)*(optional)*

Directions   *Preheat oven to 300 degrees.*

1. In a food processor, process cashews to small pieces, but not powder. Place into a medium-sized bowl. Process almond slices, walnut pieces, pecan pieces, and dates, one at a time, in the same manner.
2. Add the honey and rice bran to the nut mixture. Stir to combine.
3. Transfer to a cookie sheet, spreading out evenly. Toast in a 300-degree oven for 20-30 minutes or until lightly browned.
4. Return to bowl. Add the golden raisins, raisins, and coconut. Stir to combine. Allow to cool.

Makes 6 cups. Store in snack size bags in the refrigerator for one month or the freezer for three months.

Variation: Replace some of the nuts with peanuts, if allowed. For other nut allergies, remove the nut and replace with one that does not cause a reaction. Add roasted soy nuts instead of peanuts for a similar flavor. Add ½ cup sweetened chocolate or carob chips after cooling, if desired.

---

* Read the ingredients carefully. Sometimes flour is used to prevent dates from sticking to each other. Be sure to select a gluten-free variety.

Popcorn

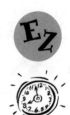

Ingredients

2 tablespoons vegetable oil
1 cup popcorn kernels

Directions

1. In a large saucepan, heat the oil until hot. (A drop of water will crackle when it is hot enough.) Be careful not to burn the oil.
2. Add the popcorn kernels and cover.
3. Shake the pan continuously slightly above the burner until the first kernel pops. Then shake constantly until the popping slows to one pop every one or two seconds. Remove from heat.
4. Pour the popcorn into a bowl and add salt or one of the toppings listed below. Removing the unpopped kernels before adding the topping of your choice makes for a more pleasant eating experience but is optional.

Makes 9 to 10 cups popcorn.

Buttered popcorn: Melt 3 tablespoons of margarine or butter in the same saucepan. Drizzle over the popcorn, add a dash of salt, and toss.

Caramel corn: In the same saucepan, heat 1½ tablespoons of margarine or butter, ½ cup packed brown sugar, 2 tablespoons half-and-half or nondairy creamer, and 1 tablespoon of light corn syrup to boiling, stirring occasionally. Reduce heat and simmer for one minute, stirring constantly. Drizzle over the popcorn and toss well.

Parmesan popcorn: Prepare buttered popcorn above, omitting salt. Sprinkle ½ cup grated Parmesan cheese and toss.

Italian popcorn: In the same saucepan, melt ¼ cup margarine or butter. Remove from heat. Add ½ cup Parmesan cheese, ¼ teaspoon garlic salt, ½ teaspoon dried and crushed oregano, and ½ teaspoon dried and crushed basil. Drizzle over popcorn and toss.

Mexican popcorn: In the same saucepan, melt 3 tablespoons of margarine or butter. Remove from heat. Add ¼ teaspoon mild chili powder. Drizzle over popcorn and toss.

Sport Drink

Here is a natural electrolyte replacement.
Can be used for sports or during an illness.

Ingredients

½ gallon apple juice
½ gallon white grape juice
1 2-liter bottle of seltzer water (optional)

Directions

1. In a one-gallon jar or pitcher, combine the apple juice and the white grape juice.
2. To serve, fill a glass half-full with the juice and add the seltzer water and ice to fill. (Can also be served without the seltzer water, but you lose the fun fizz.)

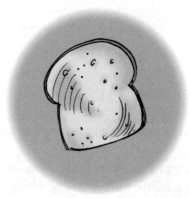

Breads

Quick Breads ❦ Yeast Breads ❦ Bread Machine

"Ask God's blessing on your work,

but don't ask Him to do it for you."

—Dame Flora Robinson

About Gluten-Free Bread

Bread is one of the basic staples, and may be one of the hardest foods to give up on a gluten-free diet.

Gluten-free breads do not have the same consistency as breads made with wheat. They tend to be more dense and crumbly. Many gluten-free types of bread available in health food stores are very hard and about as tasty as cardboard. They also come at a price, usually running fifty cents to a dollar per slice. That cost can be quite an investment if your child hates the bread.

Homemade breads, such as those made with the following recipes, are moister and softer than the gluten-free breads you can purchase. The cost to produce your own bread is a fraction of the cost of the pre-made gluten-free breads, running closer to the cost of premium wheat breads from a bakery or deli. Purchasing the baking ingredients in bulk further reduces the cost.

The following recipes for yeast and bread machine breads stand up very well to a sandwich, especially if slightly warmed. If you want an even moister, higher rising bread, you can add up to one full tablespoon of unflavored gelatin. (If you use more than one tablespoon, the bread will retain moisture when you store it, and the crust will get soggy.)

Many of the bread recipes do very well doubled. For longer shelf life, store these breads in an airtight container or zip-style bag in the refrigerator or freezer, since the recipes do not include any preservatives. You can reduce your baking efforts if you bake extra loaves of bread at one time, slice them to the desired thickness, and place a piece of waxed paper or parchment paper in between the slices. Then store the bread in a freezer zip-style bag in a deep freeze for up to three months or refrigerator freezer for up to six weeks.

The recipes may look a little complicated at first, but as you discover which breads are your favorites, they become more familiar and easier to prepare.

Gluten-free breads are a bit different from the breads around us everyday, but with a little planning, your endeavors will be well worth the time in cost and taste—not to mention the smile on your child's face.

*"The best inheritance a parent can give his children
is a few minutes of his time each day."*
—A. Battista

Quick Breads

Banana Bread

Ingredients

½ cup brown rice flour
½ cup rice flour
½ cup tapioca flour
¼ cup potato starch flour
⅔ cup sugar
2 teaspoons baking powder
1 teaspoon baking soda
1 teaspoon xanthan gum
¼ teaspoon salt
⅓ cup shortening
2 tablespoons milk
2 eggs
1 cup mashed bananas (2-3 medium)
⅓ cup chopped nuts (optional)

Directions   *Preheat oven to 375 degrees.*

1. In a large bowl, combine brown rice flour, rice flour, tapioca flour, potato starch flour, sugar, baking powder, baking soda, xanthan gum, and salt. Cut in shortening until mixture is crumbly.
2. In another bowl, combine the milk and eggs, beating slightly.
3. Add half of the milk mixture. With an electric mixer, beat to combine. Add half the mashed banana and beat to combine. Repeat with remaining milk mixture and banana, beating between additions.
4. Beat the batter on medium speed for three minutes. Add nuts, if desired, and combine.
5. Pour into a greased loaf pan or three greased mini-loaf pans. Bake at 375 degrees for 55-60 minutes for a large loaf or 40-50 minutes for mini-loaves or until a toothpick inserted near the center of the loaf comes out clean.
6. Cool for 10 minutes on wire rack. Remove from pan. Cool completely on wire rack before slicing.
7. Slice and store in an air-tight container or zip-style bag in the refrigerator for a week to ten days.

Makes 16 servings.

Biscuits Supreme

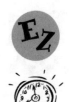

Ingredients

1 cup rice flour
⅔ cup potato starch flour
⅓ cup tapioca flour
1 tablespoon baking powder
1 teaspoon baking soda
½ teaspoon xanthan gum
2 teaspoons sugar
¼ teaspoon salt
⅓ cup margarine or butter
⅔ cup milk or substitute

Directions

Preheat oven to 450 degrees.

1. In a large bowl, combine rice flour, potato starch flour, tapioca flour, baking powder, baking soda, xanthan gum, sugar, salt, and margarine until crumbly. Make a well by pushing the dry ingredients to the sides of the bowl.
2. Add the milk all at once. Mix until completely moistened but do not over mix. The batter will be slightly lumpy.
3. Drop by heaping tablespoonfuls onto a greased cookie sheet. Bake in 450-degree oven for 10-12 minutes or until lightly browned.

Makes 15 biscuits.

Buttermilk Biscuits

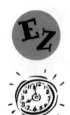

Ingredients

1½ cups rice flour
⅓ cup potato starch flour
3 tablespoons tapioca flour
1 tablespoon baking powder
¼ teaspoon baking soda
2 teaspoons sugar
2 teaspoons Cream of Tartar
¼ teaspoon salt
1 teaspoon xanthan gum
2½ teaspoons powdered buttermilk
½ cup margarine or butter, softened
½ cup water
1 egg, beaten

Directions

Preheat oven to 450 degrees.

1. In a bowl, combine rice flour, potato starch flour, tapioca flour, baking powder, baking soda, sugar, Cream of Tartar, salt, xanthan gum, and powdered buttermilk.
2. Cut in the margarine with a pastry blender or an electric mixer on low. Make a well in the center and add the water and egg all at once.
3. Mix well until moistened and combined.
4. Drop by spoonfuls onto a greased cookie sheet. Bake in a 450-degree oven for 10-12 minutes, or until golden.

Makes 12 biscuits.

Corn Bread

Ingredients

1 cup corn meal
½ cup rice flour
½ cup tapioca flour
1 teaspoon xanthan gum
2 tablespoons sugar
1 tablespoon baking powder
½ teaspoon salt
2 eggs
1 cup milk
¼ cup oil

Directions

Preheat oven to 425 degrees.

1. In a medium-sized bowl, combine the corn meal, rice flour, tapioca flour, xanthan gum, sugar, baking powder, and salt.
2. In a small bowl, beat the eggs, milk, and oil slightly to combine.
3. Add the egg mixture to the flour mixture and stir until the batter is smooth. Do not overbeat.
4. Pour into a greased 9 x 9 x 2-inch baking pan. Bake at 425 degrees for 20-25 minutes or until golden brown, and toothpick inserted near center comes out clean.

Makes 9 servings.

Corn Bread Mini-Loaf: Prepare as above, except pour into two greased 9 x 5 x 3-inch loaf pans. Bake for 20-25 minutes or until golden brown. Makes 8 servings.

Corn Bread Muffins: Prepare as above, except spoon the batter into greased muffin pans, filling ⅔ full. Bake as above for 12-15 minutes or until golden brown. Makes 12 muffins.

Garlic Biscuits

Ingredients

1 cup rice flour
⅔ cup potato starch flour
⅓ cup tapioca flour
1 tablespoon baking powder
1 teaspoon baking soda
½ teaspoon xanthan gum
2 teaspoons sugar
¼ teaspoon salt
1 tablespoon dried parsley, crushed
1-2 cloves garlic, minced
⅓ cup margarine or butter
⅔ cup milk or substitute

Directions

Preheat oven to 450 degrees.

1. In a large bowl, combine rice flour, potato starch flour, tapioca flour, baking powder, baking soda, xanthan gum, sugar, salt, parsley, garlic, and margarine until crumbly.
2. Make a well by pushing the dry ingredients to the sides of the bowl. Add the milk all at once. Mix until completely moistened but do not over mix. (Batter will be lumpy.)
3. Drop by heaping tablespoonfuls onto a greased cookie sheet. Bake at 450 degrees for 10-12 minutes or until lightly browned.

Makes 15 biscuits.

Mock Flour Tortillas

Ingredients

½ cup brown rice flour
½ cup rice flour
½ cup potato starch flour
½ cup tapioca flour
1 tablespoon xanthan gum
1 teaspoon salt
3 tablespoons shortening
¾ cup hot water

Directions

1. In a large bowl, combine the brown rice flour, rice flour, potato starch flour, tapioca flour, xanthan gum, and salt. Add shortening and cut in with a pastry blender or two knifes until crumbly like breadcrumbs.
2. Add water and stir with a spoon. Form into a ball with hands.
3. Divide the dough into 12 balls.
4. Press with a tortilla press or a rolling pin, with lightly oiled plastic wrap on both the top and the bottom of the dough.
5. Preheat ungreased griddle to about 400 degrees, if electric, or until a droplet of water dropped on the griddle crackles.
6. Cook tortillas until bubbles form and the bottoms are lightly browned. Turn and cook the other side.

Makes 12 tortillas

Zucchini Bread

■■■■■■■■■■■■■■■■■■■■■■■■■■■■■■
A moist bread that looks and tastes like the wheat variety!

Ingredients

½ cup raisins
¼ cup water
½ cup light bean flour (or brown rice flour or soy flour)
½ cup tapioca flour
½ cup rice flour
1 teaspoon baking soda
½ teaspoon baking powder
1 teaspoon xanthan gum
¾ teaspoon salt
1½ teaspoons ground cinnamon
¼ teaspoon ground nutmeg
1 egg
1 cup shredded, unpeeled zucchini
1½ teaspoons vanilla
⅓ cup cooking oil
1 cup sugar
½ cup chopped walnuts *(optional)*
¼ teaspoon finely shredded lemon peel

Directions   *Preheat oven to 350 degrees.*

1. In a small pan, boil the raisins and water for one minute. Drain, reserving the water. Allow the raisins to cool.
2. In a medium bowl, sift together the bean flour, tapioca flour, rice flour, baking soda, baking powder, xanthan gum, salt, cinnamon, and nutmeg. Set aside.
3. In a large bowl, beat the egg. Add the zucchini and mix well. Add the vanilla, oil, sugar, and half of the flour mixture. Beat well. Add the raisins, the reserved water from the raisins, walnuts (if desired), lemon peel, and the remainder of the flour mixture. Mix well.
4. Pour the batter into a greased 8 x 4 x 2-inch loaf pan. Bake in a 350-degree oven for 55-60 minutes or until a toothpick inserted near the center of the loaf comes out clean.

5. Cool on a wire rack for 10 minutes. Remove the bread from the pan and cool completely on a wire rack before slicing.

Makes 1 loaf.

Note: Store the sliced bread in plastic wrap or in a large zip-style bag in the refrigerator.

Apple Bread: Prepare as above, substituting shredded apple for the zucchini.

Applesauce Bread: Prepare as above, substituting 1 cup drained applesauce for the zucchini.

*"Non-cooks think it's silly to invest two hours' work
in two minutes' enjoyment; but if cooking
is evanescent, so is the ballet."*
—Julia Child

Yeast Breads

Almond Bread

▪▪▪▪▪▪▪▪▪▪▪▪▪▪▪▪▪▪▪▪▪▪▪▪▪▪

Similar in taste and texture to oatmeal bread.

Ingredients

1½ cups rice flour
1 cup tapioca flour
⅓ cup packed brown sugar
1 tablespoon xanthan gum
½ teaspoon salt
1 tablespoon unflavored gelatin (optional)
2¼ teaspoons (1 package) dry yeast
1½ cups (6-ounce package) sliced almonds
3 tablespoons shortening
1 cup water
1 teaspoon rice vinegar
3 large eggs

Directions

1. In a large bowl, combine rice flour, tapioca flour, brown sugar, xanthan gum, salt, gelatin (if used), and yeast.
2. Preheat oven to 200 degrees.
3. Place the almond slices in a zip-style bag, squeeze out the air, and seal. Using a rolling pin, crush the almonds until they are the size of oatmeal. Reserve 2 tablespoons of almonds. Add remaining almonds to the flour mixture. Add the shortening and combine until crumbly.
4. Heat the water to 120 to 130 degrees on a candy thermometer. With an electric mixer on low (or a heavy-duty mixer on slow), add the water slowly to the dry ingredients. Add the vinegar and eggs one at a time. Beat on high-speed of the electric mixer for three minutes (or medium in a heavy-duty mixer).
5. Pour the dough into two greased loaf pans. Sprinkle with reserved almonds. Put the filled pans into the pre-heated oven; turn the oven off. Let the dough rise until doubled, about 45 to 60 minutes.
6. Turn oven on (with bread still in it) to 375 degrees and bake for 30 to 35 minutes until the loaves are browned and a toothpick inserted

near the center comes out clean. (Cover both loaves with foil halfway through bake time, if needed to prevent over-browning.)

7. Remove loaves from the oven and cool on a wire rack for 10 minutes. Remove the bread from the pans and cool completely on the wire rack before slicing.

Makes 2 loaves.

Dinner Rolls: Prepare as above, except spoon dough into greased muffin tins, about half full. Sprinkle with the remaining almonds. Bake for 15-20 minutes, or until rolls test done as above. Cool for 10 minutes, then remove from muffin pan. Serve warm. Makes about 36 rolls.

Bean Potato Bread

*This bread adds proteins to the starches for a more complete food product.
It is especially good if your child doesn't have enough protein in his diet.*

Ingredients

1 cup light bean flour*
1 cup rice flour
1 cup tapioca flour
½ cup potato flour (**not** starch)
1 tablespoon xanthan gum
1½ teaspoons salt
1 teaspoon unflavored gelatin
⅓ cup packed brown sugar
2¼ teaspoons (one package) dry yeast
¼ cup (½ stick) margarine or butter
2 cups milk or milk substitute
1 teaspoon rice or apple vinegar
3 large eggs or ¾ cup egg substitute

Directions

1. Combine bean, rice, tapioca, and potato flours, xanthan gum, salt, unflavored gelatin, brown sugar, and yeast in a large mixing bowl (or the large bowl of a heavy-duty mixer with a flat beater).
2. Preheat oven to 200 degrees.
3. Melt the margarine in the milk until it is 120-130 degrees on a candy thermometer (do not scald).
4. With an electric mixer on low speed (or a heavy-duty mixer on slow), slowly add the milk/margarine mixture to the dry ingredients. Add the vinegar and the eggs, one at a time. Beat at highest speed of the mixer for three minutes (or medium in a heavy-duty mixer). The dough will look like thick cake batter.
5. Pour the dough into two greased loaf pans. Put the filled pans into the pre-heated oven; turn the oven off. Let the dough rise until doubled, about 45 to 60 minutes.

6. Turn oven on (with bread still in it) to 375 degrees and bake for 35 to 40 minutes until the loaves are golden and a toothpick inserted near the center comes out clean. (Cover both loaves with foil halfway through bake time, if needed, to prevent over-browning.)
7. Remove loaves from oven and cool on a wire rack for 10 minutes. Remove the bread from the pans and cool completely on the wire rack before slicing. Makes 2 loaves.

Note: Substitute instant mashed potato flakes for the potato flour, if desired. (Light bean flour can be substituted with brown rice flour, or rice flour, if desired. Protein levels will be changed.)

---

*   Garfava, full fat soy, or garbanzo bean flour

Classic White Bread

This bread is my son's favorite because it reminds him of traditional white (wheat-type) bread.

Ingredients

2 cups rice flour
1 cup potato starch flour
½ cup tapioca flour
2 tablespoons sugar
1 tablespoon xanthan gum
1½ teaspoons salt
½ cup nonfat dry milk
2¼ teaspoons (1 package) dry yeast
1 teaspoon unflavored gelatin (optional)
1½ cups water
2 tablespoons margarine or butter
1 teaspoon rice vinegar
3 large eggs

Directions

1. Combine rice, potato starch, and tapioca flours, sugar, xanthan gum, salt, milk powder, yeast, and unflavored gelatin in a large mixing bowl (or the large bowl of a heavy-duty mixer with a flat beater).
2. Preheat oven to 200 degrees.
3. Melt the margarine in the water until the water is 120-130 degrees on a candy thermometer.
4. With an electric mixer on low speed (or a heavy-duty mixer on slow), slowly add the water/margarine mixture to the dry ingredients. Add the vinegar and the eggs, one at a time. Beat at highest speed of the mixer for three minutes (or medium in a heavy-duty mixer). The dough will look like thick cake batter.
5. Pour the dough into two greased loaf pans. Put the filled pans into the pre-heated oven; turn the oven off. Let the dough rise until doubled, about 45 to 60 minutes.
6. Turn oven on (with bread still in it) to 375 degrees and bake for 35 to

40 minutes until the loaves are golden and a toothpick inserted near the center comes out clean. (Cover both loaves with foil halfway through bake time, if needed, to prevent over-browning.)

7. Remove loaves from oven and cool on a wire rack for 10 minutes. Remove the bread from the pans and cool completely on the wire rack before slicing.

Makes 2 loaves.

To Prepare without Milk: Replace water with milk substitute (like Mocha Mix®), delete the powdered milk, and use shortening or milk-free margarine (like Nucoa®). Continue as above.

Garlic Toast

Ingredients

6 slices of gluten-free bread, ½ -1 inch thick
¼ cup butter or margarine
¼ teaspoon garlic powder
¼ teaspoon dried oregano, crushed
1 tablespoon grated Parmesan cheese

Directions

1. Toast the bread in a toaster or broil for 2 minutes in the oven.
2. Meanwhile, melt the butter in a small pan on the stovetop or in a microwavable bowl in the microwave.
3. Add the garlic and oregano to the melted butter.
4. Brush the butter mixture on the top of the toasted bread slices.
5. Sprinkle with Parmesan cheese.

Makes 6 1-slice servings

Hamburger Buns

Directions

1. Prepare a yeast bread recipe as directed. (Any recipes from this section of the book work well.)
2. Preheat oven to 200 degrees.
3. Spoon dough into greased tart-sized pie tins about ⅓ full. (Disposable tart pans, English muffin rings, glass custard cups, large muffin pans, or tuna fish cans with the tops and the bottoms removed, thoroughly cleaned, can be used as hamburger molds as well.) Sprinkle with sesame seeds, if desired.
4. Put the filled molds into the preheated oven; turn the oven off. Let the dough rise until doubled, about 30-45 minutes.
5. Turn the oven on (with the buns still in it) to 375 degrees and bake for 25-30 minutes, or until a toothpick inserted near the center comes out clean.
6. Remove the buns from the oven to cool on a wire rack for 10 minutes.
7. Remove the buns from the molds. Cool completely.
8. Slice each bun in half and insert a piece of waxed paper between the slices.
9. Store buns in a labeled, dated, freezer zip-style bag for up to four months in the freezer or six months in a deep-freezer.

Makes 12 hamburger buns.

Hot Dog Buns

Directions

1. Prepare a yeast bread recipe as directed. (Any yeast bread or bread machine recipe in the book works well.)
2. Preheat oven to 200 degrees.
3. Make hot dog molds as follows:

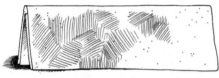
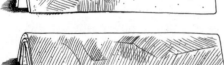
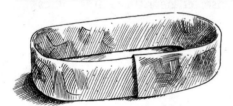

   a. Tear off a strip of foil about 12 inches long.
   b. Fold in half to 6 inches long.
   c. Fold in half again to 3 inches long, and in half again until the foil is a thick strip about 1½ inches tall.
   d. Bring ends of the foil strip together (as if making a paper chain), tucking one end into the folds of the other end to connect. Grease well.
   e. Shape the mold into an oblong about 2½ inches wide at the center and place on a well-greased cookie sheet. Repeat 11 more times.
4. Spoon dough into the molds. Put the cookie sheet with the filled molds into the preheated oven; turn the oven off. Let the dough rise until doubled, about 30-45 minutes.
5. Turn the oven on (with the buns still in it) to 375 degrees and bake for 25-30 minutes, or until a toothpick inserted near the center comes out clean.
6. Remove the buns from the oven to cool on a wire rack for 10 minutes.
7. Remove the buns from the molds. Cool completely.
8. Slice each bun in half and insert a piece of waxed paper between the slices.
9. Store buns in a labeled, dated, freezer zip-style bag for up to four months in the freezer or six months in a deep-freezer.

Makes 12 hot dog buns.

Mock Rye Bread

Ingredients

2 cups brown rice flour
1 cup tapioca flour
½ cup potato starch flour
1 tablespoon xanthan gum
1½ teaspoons salt
⅔ cup dry milk
1 teaspoon unflavored gelatin
2¼ teaspoons (one package) dry yeast
3 tablespoons molasses
1½ teaspoons sugar
½ square (½ ounce) unsweetened baking chocolate, cut up
1 tablespoon vinegar
¼ cup shortening
1¼ cup liquid coffee (brewed or instant)
1 tablespoon caraway seeds
½ teaspoon fennel seed, crushed
3 large eggs

Directions

1. In a large bowl, combine brown rice flour, tapioca flour, potato starch flour, xanthan gum, salt, dry milk, unflavored gelatin, and dry yeast.
2. In a saucepan, combine molasses, sugar, chocolate, vinegar, and shortening and heat until the chocolate melts. Add the coffee and heat until the liquid is 120-130 degrees on a candy thermometer. Remove from heat.
3. Preheat oven to 200 degrees.
4. With an electric mixer on low speed (or a heavy-duty mixer on slow), slowly add the chocolate mixture to the dry ingredients, scraping the sides of the bowl occasionally. Beat one minute.
5. Add the caraway and fennel. Add the eggs, one at a time, beating well after each addition. Beat at highest speed of the mixer for three

minutes (or medium in a heavy-duty mixer.) The dough will look like thick cake batter.

6. Pour the dough into two greased loaf pans. Put the filled pans into the pre-heated oven; turn the oven off. Let the dough rise until doubled, about 45 to 60 minutes.

7. Turn oven on (with bread still in it) to 375 degrees and bake for 30 to 35 minutes until the loaves are browned and a toothpick inserted near the center comes out clean. (Cover both loaves with foil halfway through bake time, if needed, to prevent over-browning.)

8. Remove loaves from oven and cool on a wire rack for 10 minutes. Remove the bread from the pans and cool completely on the wire rack before slicing.

Makes 2 loaves.

To Prepare without Milk: Replace water with milk substitute (like Mocha Mix®), omit the powdered milk, and use shortening or milk-free margarine (like Nucoa®). Continue as above.

Dinner Rolls: Prepare as above, except spoon dough into greased muffin tins, about half full. Bake for 15-20 minutes, or until rolls test done as above. Cool for 10 minutes; remove from muffin pan. Serve warm. Makes about 36 rolls.

Rice Tapioca Bread

Ingredients

2 cups rice flour
1½ cups tapioca flour
¼ cup packed brown sugar
1 tablespoon xanthan gum
1 teaspoon unflavored gelatin (optional)
1½ teaspoons salt
⅔ cup nonfat non-instant dry milk powder
2¼ teaspoons (one package) dry yeast
¼ cup shortening, margarine, or butter
1⅓ cups water
1 teaspoon rice vinegar
3 large eggs

Directions

1. Combine rice flour, tapioca flour, brown sugar, xanthan gum, unflavored gelatin, salt, milk powder, yeast, and shortening in a large mixing bowl (or the large bowl of a heavy-duty mixer with a flat beater). Mix until crumbly—about 1 minute.
2. Preheat oven to 200 degrees.
3. Heat the water to 120-130 degrees on a candy thermometer.
4. With an electric mixer on low speed (or a heavy-duty mixer on slow), slowly add the water to the dry ingredients. Add the vinegar and the eggs, one at a time. Beat at highest speed of the mixer for three minutes (or medium in a heavy-duty mixer). The dough will look like thick cake batter.
5. Pour the dough into two greased loaf pans. Put the filled pans into the pre-heated oven; turn the oven off. Let the dough rise until doubled, about 45 to 60 minutes.
6. Turn oven on (with bread still in it) to 375 degrees and bake for 35 to 40 minutes until the loaves are golden and a toothpick inserted near the center comes out clean. (Cover both loaves with foil halfway through bake time, if needed, to prevent over-browning.)

7. Remove loaves from oven and cool on a wire rack for 10 minutes. Remove the bread from the pans and cool completely on the wire rack before slicing.

Makes 2 loaves.

To Prepare without Milk: Replace water with milk substitute (like Mocha Mix®), omit the powdered milk, and use shortening or milk-free margarine (like Nucoa®). Continue as above.

Dinner Rolls: Prepare as above, except spoon dough into greased muffin pans, about half full. Bake for 20-25 minutes, or until rolls test done as described above. Cool for 10 minutes; remove from muffin pan. Serve warm. Makes about 36 rolls.

Cinnamon Nut Bread: Prepare as above through Step 4. In a small bowl combine ⅓ cup brown sugar, ⅓ cup finely chopped pecans, walnuts, almonds, or other nut, and 1 teaspoon ground cinnamon. Sprinkle 1½ tablespoons of the sugar mixture on the bottom of each of the greased loaf pans. Fill the loaf pans ¼ full and sprinkle half of the remaining sugar mixture on the batter. Fill the loaf pans with the remaining batter (about half full.) Sprinkle with the remaining sugar mixture. Rise and bake as above. Serve warm with a powdered sugar glaze, if desired. Makes 2 loaves.

(Powdered sugar glaze: Mix one cup of sifted powdered sugar, one tablespoon of milk or water, and ¼ teaspoon pure vanilla extract. Stir in one teaspoon milk or water at a time until it is of drizzling consistency. Drizzle ½ of the glaze over each loaf.)

Cinnamon Nut Rolls: Prepare as described for cinnamon nut bread, except use well-greased muffin pans instead of loaf pans. Rise and bake as for dinner rolls above. Makes 36 rolls.

Sesame Bread

Ingredients

2 cups rice flour
1 cup potato starch flour
½ cup tapioca flour
2 tablespoons sugar
1 tablespoon xanthan gum
1½ teaspoons salt
½ cup nonfat dry milk
2¼ teaspoons (1 package) dry yeast
1 teaspoon unflavored gelatin (optional)
¼ cup sesame seeds
1¾ cups water
¼ cup margarine or butter
1 teaspoon rice vinegar
3 large eggs

Directions

1. Combine rice, potato starch, and tapioca flours, sugar, xanthan gum, salt, milk powder, yeast, and unflavored gelatin in a large mixing bowl (or the large bowl of a heavy-duty mixer with a flat beater).
2. Reserve 3 tablespoons sesame seeds and set aside. Add remaining sesame seeds to flour mixture and combine.
3. Preheat oven to 200 degrees.
4. Melt the margarine in the water until the water is 120-130 degrees on a candy thermometer.
5. With an electric mixer on low speed (or a heavy-duty mixer on slow), slowly add the water/margarine mixture to the dry ingredients. Add the vinegar and the eggs, one at a time. Beat at highest speed of the mixer for three minutes (or medium on the heavy-duty mixer).The dough will look like thick cake batter.
6. Pour the dough into two greased loaf pans. Sprinkle each loaf with 1½ tablespoons reserved sesame seeds. Put the filled pans into the

pre-heated oven; turn the oven off. Let the dough rise until doubled, about 45 to 60 minutes.

7. Turn oven on (with bread still in it) to 375 degrees and bake for 35 to 40 minutes until the loaves are golden and a toothpick inserted near the center comes out clean. (Cover both loaves with foil halfway through bake time, if needed, to prevent over-browning.)

8. Remove loaves from oven and cool on a wire rack for 10 minutes. Remove the bread from the pans and cool completely on the wire rack before slicing.

Makes 2 loaves.

To Prepare without Milk: Replace water with milk substitute (like Mocha Mix®), omit the powdered milk, and use shortening or milk-free margarine (like Nucoa®). Continue as above.

Whole Grain Brown Rice Bread

Ingredients

1 cup whole brown rice
2 cups water
2 cups brown rice flour
1½ cups tapioca flour
¼ cup packed brown sugar
1 tablespoon xanthan gum
1 teaspoon salt
⅔ cup dry milk powder
2¼ teaspoons (one package) dry yeast
¼ cup margarine, butter, or shortening
1¼ cups water
1 teaspoon rice or apple cider vinegar
3 large eggs, room temperature

Directions

1. In a saucepan, combine the whole grain rice and the 2 cups of water. Bring to a boil. Cover and reduce heat. Simmer for 40 minutes or until all the water is absorbed. Remove from heat and set aside.
2. Combine brown rice flour, tapioca flour, sugar, xanthan gum, salt, milk powder, yeast, and margarine in a large mixing bowl (or the large bowl of a heavy-duty mixer with a flat beater). Combine until crumbly—about 1 minute.
3. Preheat oven to 200 degrees.
4. Heat the water to 120-130 degrees on a candy thermometer.
5. With an electric mixer on low speed (or a heavy-duty mixer on slow) slowly add the water to the dry ingredients. Add the cooked brown rice. Add the vinegar and the eggs, one at a time. Beat at highest speed of the mixer for three minutes (or medium in a heavy-duty mixer). The dough will look like thick cake batter.
6. Pour the dough into two greased loaf pans. Put the filled pans into the pre-heated oven; turn the oven off. Let the dough rise until doubled, about 45 to 60 minutes.

7. Turn oven on (with bread still in it) to 375 degrees and bake for 35 to 40 minutes or until the loaves are golden and a toothpick inserted near the center comes out clean. (Cover both loaves with foil halfway through bake time, if needed, to prevent over-browning.)
8. Remove loaves from oven and cool on a wire rack for 10 minutes. Remove the bread from the pans and cool completely on the wire rack before slicing.

Makes 2 loaves.

To Prepare without Milk: Replace water with milk substitute (like Mocha Mix®), omit the powdered milk, and use shortening or milk-free margarine (like Nucoa®). Continue as above.

Dinner Rolls: Prepare as above, except spoon dough into greased muffin tins, about half full. Bake for 20-25 minutes, or until rolls test done as described above. Cool for 10 minutes. Remove from muffin pan. Serve warm. Makes 34-36 rolls.

"Motivation is what gets you started.
Habit is what keeps you going."
—Jim Ryan

Bread Machine

The bread machine recipes in this section were reprinted with permission from Red Star® Yeast and Products from "Gluten-Free Recipes for Your Bread Machine" in the Red Star® Yeast & Products brochure.

Brown & White Bread

Wet Ingredients

3 large eggs, lightly beaten
1 teaspoon cider vinegar
3 tablespoons canola oil
1½ cups plus 2 tablespoons water

Dry Ingredients

2¼ cups white rice flour
1 cup brown rice flour
1½ teaspoons xanthan gum
3 tablespoons sugar
1½ teaspoons salt
1 tablespoon egg replacer, optional
½ cup dry milk
2¼ teaspoons (one package) RED STAR® Active Dry Yeast

Bread Machine Directions

1. Combine the wet ingredients; pour carefully into the baking pan.
2. Measure the dry ingredients into a bowl; mix thoroughly to blend. Add to the baking pan. Carefully seat the bread pan in the bread maker.
3. Select NORMAL/WHITE cycle; start the machine.
4. After the mixing action begins, help mix any unmixed ingredients into the dough with a rubber spatula, keeping to the edges and the top of pan to prevent interference with the paddle. (Dough for gluten-free bread is similar to that of quick breads: stiffer than cake batter, but not as stiff as cookie dough. If the dough appears too dry, add liquid, one tablespoon at a time, to achieve a consistency that allows the bread machine to mix by itself.)
5. Remove pan from the machine as soon as the bake cycle is complete. Invert pan and gently shake to remove the bread. Cool completely, upright on rack, before slicing.

Conventional Directions

1. Combine the liquid ingredients in a mixing bowl and whisk together.
2. Combine all the dry ingredients in the bowl of a heavy-duty mixer or a large mixing bowl and whisk together.
3. Using a heavy-duty mixer on slow, add the wet ingredients to the dry ingredients. (Or mix on low with a hand-held electric mixer.)
4. Beat the batter for about 10 minutes on medium speed.
5. Pour batter into a large, greased bread pan.
6. Allow batter to rise until nearly doubled, about 1 hour.
7. Bake at 375 degrees for 45-60 minutes; use a toothpick to check for doneness.
8. Remove loaf from pan as soon as baking is complete. Invert pan and gently shake to remove the bread. Cool completely on a rack before slicing.

Chickpea Bread

Wet Ingredients

3 large eggs, lightly beaten
1 teaspoon cider vinegar
3 tablespoons olive oil
1⅓ cups water
¼ teaspoon gluten-free maple flavoring extract (optional)

Dry Ingredients

1 cup chickpea flour
1 cup brown or white rice flour
1 cup tapioca flour
½ cup cornstarch
4 teaspoons xanthan gum
3 tablespoons brown sugar
1½ teaspoons salt
1 tablespoon egg replacer (optional)
½ cup dry milk
2¼ teaspoons (one package) RED STAR® Active Dry Yeast

Bread Machine Directions

1. Combine the wet ingredients; pour carefully into the baking pan.
2. Measure the dry ingredients into a bowl; mix thoroughly to blend. Add to the baking pan. Carefully seat the bread pan in the bread maker.
3. Select NORMAL/WHITE cycle; start the machine.
4. After the mixing action begins, help mix any unmixed ingredients into the dough with a rubber spatula, keeping to the edges and the top of pan to prevent interference with the paddle. (Dough for gluten-free bread is similar to that of quick breads: stiffer than cake batter, but not as stiff as cookie dough. If the dough appears too dry, add liquid, one tablespoon at a time, to achieve a consistency that allows the bread machine to mix by itself.)

5. Remove pan from the machine as soon as the bake cycle is complete. Invert pan and gently shake to remove the bread. Cool completely, upright on rack, before slicing.

Conventional Directions

1. Combine the liquid ingredients in a mixing bowl and whisk together.
2. Combine all the dry ingredients in the bowl of a heavy-duty mixer or a large mixing bowl and whisk together.
3. Using a heavy-duty mixer on slow, add the wet ingredients to the dry ingredients. (Or mix on low with a hand-held electric mixer.)
4. Beat the batter for about 10 minutes on medium speed.
5. Pour batter into a large, greased bread pan.
6. Allow batter to rise until nearly doubled, about 1 hour.
7. Bake at 375 degrees for 45-60 minutes; use a toothpick to check for doneness.
8. Remove loaf from pan as soon as baking is complete. Invert pan and gently shake to remove the bread. Cool completely, on a rack, before slicing.

Delicate Buttermilk Bread

Wet Ingredients

3 large eggs, lightly beaten
¼ cup canola oil or melted butter
1¼ cups plus 2 tablespoons water

Dry Ingredients

2 cups white rice flour
½ cup potato starch flour
½ cup tapioca flour
⅓ cup cornstarch
1 tablespoon xanthan gum
2 tablespoons sugar
1½ teaspoons salt
1 tablespoon egg replacer (optional)
½ cup powdered milk
2¼ teaspoons (1 package) RED STAR® Active Dry Yeast

Bread Machine Directions

1. Combine the wet ingredients; pour carefully into the baking pan.
2. Measure the dry ingredients into a bowl; mix thoroughly to blend. Add to the baking pan. Carefully seat the bread pan in the bread maker.
3. Select NORMAL/WHITE cycle; start the machine.
4. After the mixing action begins, help mix any unmixed ingredients into the dough with a rubber spatula, keeping to the edges and the top of pan to prevent interference with the paddle. (Dough for gluten-free bread is similar to that of quick breads: stiffer than cake batter, but not as stiff as cookie dough. If the dough appears too dry, add liquid, one tablespoon at a time, to achieve a consistency that allows the bread machine to mix by itself.)
5. Remove pan from the machine as soon as the bake cycle is complete. Invert pan and gently shake to remove the bread. Cool completely, upright on rack, before slicing.

Conventional Directions

1. Combine the liquid ingredients in a mixing bowl and whisk together.
2. Combine all the dry ingredients in the bowl of a heavy-duty mixer or a large mixing bowl and whisk together.
3. Using a heavy-duty mixer on slow, add the wet ingredients to the dry ingredients. (Or mix on low with a hand-held electric mixer.)
4. Beat the batter for about 10 minutes on medium speed.
5. Pour batter into a large, greased bread pan.
6. Allow batter to rise until nearly doubled, about 1 hour.
7. Bake at 375 degrees for 45-60 minutes; use a toothpick to check for doneness.
8. Remove loaf from pan as soon as baking is complete. Invert pan and gently shake to remove the bread. Cool completely, on a rack, before slicing.

Brown Rice & Cranberry Bread

Wet Ingredients

    3 large eggs, lightly beaten
    1 teaspoon cider vinegar
    3 tablespoons canola oil
    1½ cups water

Dry Ingredients

    3 cups brown rice flour
    ¼ cup soy flour
    1 tablespoon xanthan gum
    3 tablespoons sugar
    1½ teaspoons salt
    1 tablespoon egg replacer (optional)
    ½ cup dry milk
    ⅔ cup dried cranberries
    2¼ teaspoons (1 package) RED STAR® Active Dry Yeast

Bread Machine Directions

1. Combine the wet ingredients; pour carefully into the baking pan.
2. Measure the dry ingredients into a bowl; mix thoroughly to blend. Add to the baking pan. Carefully seat the bread pan in the bread maker.
3. Select NORMAL/WHITE cycle; start the machine.
4. After the mixing action begins, help mix any unmixed ingredients into the dough with a rubber spatula, keeping to the edges and the top of pan to prevent interference with the paddle. (Dough for gluten-free bread is similar to that of quick breads: stiffer than cake batter, but not as stiff as cookie dough. If the dough appears too dry, add liquid, one tablespoon at a time, to achieve a consistency that allows the bread machine to mix by itself.)

5. Remove pan from the machine as soon as the bake cycle is complete. Invert pan and gently shake to remove the bread. Cool completely, upright on rack, before slicing.

Conventional Directions

1. Combine the liquid ingredients in a mixing bowl and whisk together.
2. Combine all the dry ingredients in the bowl of a heavy-duty mixer or a large mixing bowl and whisk together.
3. Using a heavy-duty mixer on slow, add the wet ingredients to the dry ingredients. (Or mix on low with a hand-held electric mixer.)
4. Beat the batter for about 10 minutes on medium speed.
5. Pour batter into a large, greased bread pan.
6. Allow batter to rise until nearly doubled, about 1 hour.
7. Bake at 375 degrees for 45-60 minutes; use a toothpick to check for doneness.
8. Remove loaf from pan as soon as baking is complete. Invert pan and gently shake to remove the bread. Cool completely, on a rack, before slicing.

Mock Black Russian Bread

Wet Ingredients

    3 large eggs, lightly beaten
    1 teaspoon cider vinegar
    3 tablespoons olive oil
    2 tablespoons molasses
    1⅓ cups water

Dry Ingredients

    2 cups brown rice flour
    ½ cup potato starch flour
    ½ cup tapioca flour
    ⅓ cup rice bran
    1 tablespoon xanthan gum
    3 tablespoons dark brown sugar, firmly packed
    1½ teaspoons salt
    1 tablespoon egg replacer, optional
    ½ cup dry milk
    1 teaspoon instant coffee
    4½ teaspoons unsweetened cocoa
    2 tablespoons caraway seeds
    2¼ teaspoons (1 package) RED STAR® Active Dry Yeast

Bread Machine Directions

1. Combine the wet ingredients; pour carefully into the baking pan.
2. Measure the dry ingredients into a bowl; mix thoroughly to blend. Add to the baking pan. Carefully seat the bread pan in the bread maker.
3. Select NORMAL/WHITE cycle; start the machine.
4. After the mixing action begins, help mix any unmixed ingredients into the dough with a rubber spatula, keeping to the edges and the top of pan to prevent interference with the paddle. (Dough for gluten-free bread is similar to that of quick breads: stiffer than cake batter, but not as stiff as cookie dough. If the dough appears too dry, add liquid,

one tablespoon at a time, to achieve a consistency that allows the bread machine to mix by itself.)

5. Remove pan from the machine as soon as the bake cycle is complete. Invert pan and gently shake to remove the bread. Cool completely, upright on rack, before slicing.

Conventional Directions

1. Combine the liquid ingredients in a mixing bowl and whisk together.
2. Combine all the dry ingredients in the bowl of a heavy-duty mixer or a large mixing bowl and whisk together.
3. Using a heavy-duty mixer on slow, add the wet ingredients to the dry ingredients. (Or mix on low with a hand-held electric mixer.)
4. Beat the batter for about 10 minutes on medium speed.
5. Pour batter into a large, greased bread pan.
6. Allow batter to rise until nearly doubled, about 1 hour.
7. Bake at 375 degrees for 45-60 minutes; use a toothpick to check for doneness.
8. Remove loaf from pan as soon as baking is complete. Invert pan and gently shake to remove the bread. Cool completely, on a rack, before slicing.

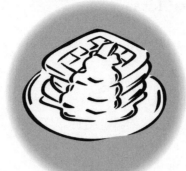

Breakfast Ideas

"To the world

you may be just one person

but to one person

you may be the world."

—Unknown

Apple Fritters

Ingredients

2 cups rice flour or brown rice flour
1 cup tapioca flour
1 cup potato starch flour
¾ cup corn meal
1 tablespoon baking powder
1 teaspoon baking soda
¼ cup sugar
1 teaspoon salt
2 beaten eggs
2 medium apples, peeled and chopped (2 cups)
2 cups milk
Shortening or cooking oil for deep fat frying
¾ cup sugar
1½ teaspoons ground cinnamon

Directions

1. In a large mixing bowl, combine rice flour, tapioca flour, potato starch flour, corn meal, baking powder, baking soda, ¼ cup sugar, and salt. Add chopped apple, milk, and beaten eggs. Stir just enough to moisten. Do not over mix.
2. Heat the shortening (at least 2 inches) in a deep fat fryer or heavy saucepan to 375 degrees on a candy thermometer.
3. Meanwhile, combine the ¾ cup sugar and ground cinnamon in a shallow bowl or pie pan. Set aside.
4. Drop batter by tablespoons, 4-5 at a time, into the hot oil. Cook for 3-4 minutes until golden brown, turning once. Drain on paper towels. Repeat.
5. Roll hot fritters in the cinnamon-sugar mixture. Serve warm.

Makes 48 fritters.

Breakfast Muffins

Ingredients

    1 cup rice flour
    ¾ cup tapioca flour
    ⅓ cup sugar
    1 tablespoon baking powder
    ¼ teaspoon salt
    ½ cup milk
    ¼ cup oil
    1 egg

Directions
Preheat oven to 350 degrees.

1. Combine rice flour, tapioca flour, sugar, baking powder, and salt in a medium bowl. Make a well by pushing ingredients to the sides of the bowl.
2. Combine milk, oil, and egg in a small bowl. Beat until well blended.
3. Add milk mixture to the flour mixture, all at once, and stir until moistened (batter will be lumpy).
4. Spoon into greased or paper-lined muffin pans, filling two-thirds full.
5. Bake 20 minutes in a 400-degree oven, or until golden and a toothpick inserted near the center comes out clean.

Makes 10 to 12 muffins.

Banana Nut Muffins: Prepare as above, except reduce milk to ¼ cup and stir in ¾ cup mashed bananas (about 2 medium) and ½ cup chopped nuts after step 3.

Banana Muffins: Prepare as for Banana Nut Muffins, omitting nuts.

Blueberry Muffins: Prepare as above, stirring in ¾ cup fresh or frozen blueberries after step 3.

Blackberry Muffins: Prepare as above, stirring in ¾ cup fresh or frozen blackberries after step 3.

Chocolate Chip Muffins: Prepare as above, stirring in ½ cup semi-sweet chocolate chips after step 3. (Do not use baking cups.)

Corn Muffins: Prepare as above, except replace the rice flour with ¾ cup corn meal. (Do not use baking cups.)

Cranberry Muffins: Prepare as above, stirring in 1 cup chopped, fresh cranberries and 2 tablespoons sugar (or ½ cup dried cranberries, like Craisins®) after step 3.

Pumpkin Muffins: Prepare as above, except add 1 teaspoon pumpkin pie spice to step 1. Then add ½ cup canned pumpkin to step 2. Add ¼ cup chopped nuts, if desired, after step 3. (Do not use baking cups.)

Buttermilk Pancakes

Ingredients

2 cups rice flour
⅓ cup tapioca flour
⅔ cup potato starch flour
3 tablespoons brown sugar
1 tablespoon baking powder
1½ teaspoons baking soda
¼ teaspoon salt
⅔ cup buttermilk powder
2 beaten eggs
2¼ cups milk
4½ teaspoons oil
1 teaspoon vanilla

Directions

1. In a large mixing bowl, combine the rice flour, tapioca flour, potato starch flour, brown sugar, baking powder, baking soda, salt, and buttermilk powder. Make a well by pushing the ingredients to the sides of the bowl.
2. In another bowl, mix the eggs, milk, and oil.
3. Add the egg mixture to the flour mixture and combine well. Do not over mix.
4. Drop by ¼ cups onto a hot griddle or pan. Cook until the pancakes are dry on the edges and bubbly. Flip and cook the other side until golden brown.

Makes 18-20 5-inch pancakes.

Note: Freeze any extra pancakes in a zip-style freezer bag. For a quick breakfast, toast or reheat in the microwave.

Cowboy Coffee Cake

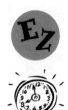

Ingredients

1 cup potato starch flour
1 cup rice flour
½ cup tapioca flour
2 cups packed brown sugar
½ teaspoon salt
⅔ cup shortening
2 teaspoons baking powder
1 teaspoon baking soda
½ teaspoon ground cinnamon
½ teaspoon ground nutmeg
1 teaspoon xanthan gum
2 teaspoons unflavored gelatin powder
½ cup raisins *(optional)*
2 beaten eggs
¾ cup milk or substitute

Directions

Preheat oven to 375 degrees.

1. In a large mixing bowl, combine the potato starch flour, rice flour, tapioca flour, brown sugar, salt, and shortening, until crumbly. Reserve ½ cup.
2. To the remaining crumbs, add baking powder, baking soda, cinnamon, nutmeg, xanthan gum, unflavored gelatin, and raisins (if used). Mix well.
3. Add the eggs and milk, mixing until moist.
4. Pour into a greased and rice-floured 9 x 13 inch baking pan.
5. Sprinkle the reserved crumbs on top.
6. Bake in a 375-degree oven for 25-30 minutes or until a toothpick inserted near the center comes out clean.
7. Serve warm with butter, if desired.

Makes 12 servings.

Crustless Quiche

Ingredients

4 eggs

1½ cups milk or substitute

¼ cup sliced green onions *(optional)*

¼ teaspoon salt

⅛ teaspoon ground pepper

⅛ teaspoon ground nutmeg

¾ cup cooked, chopped meat (chicken, ham, crabmeat) OR ½ cup crumbled bacon

2 cups (about 6 ounces) shredded cheese
    (Swiss, cheddar, Monterey Jack, Havarti)

2 tablespoons sweet rice flour

Directions   *Preheat oven to 325 degrees.*

1. Thoroughly grease a deep pie dish; set aside.
2. In a bowl, combine the eggs, milk, onion (if used), salt, pepper, and nutmeg. Stir in the meat.
3. In another bowl, combine the cheese and the sweet rice flour. Add to the egg mixture.
4. Pull out the center rack of the preheated oven and place the prepared pie pan on it. Pour the mixture carefully into the pan. Carefully push the rack back into the oven and close.
5. Cook at 325 degrees for 40-45 minutes or until a knife inserted near the center comes out clean.
6. Let stand for 10 minutes before serving.

Makes 6 servings.

Old Fashioned Cake Doughnuts

Ingredients

2 cups rice flour
1 cup tapioca flour
1 cup potato starch flour
1 teaspoon xanthan gum
2 teaspoons baking powder
1 teaspoon baking soda
1 teaspoon salt
¼ teaspoon ground cinnamon
¼ teaspoon ground nutmeg
2 eggs
⅔ cup sugar
1 teaspoon vanilla
⅔ cup milk
¼ cup margarine or butter, melted
Hot oil or shortening for frying

Directions

1. In a medium-sized bowl, combine rice flour, tapioca flour, potato starch flour, and xanthan gum.
2. In another medium-sized mixing bowl, combine 2¼ cups of the flour mix from step 1 with baking powder, baking soda, salt, ground cinnamon, and ground nutmeg.
3. In a large mixing bowl, combine the eggs, sugar, and vanilla. Add the milk and melted margarine. Add the flour mixture, from step 2, one-fourth at a time, beating with electric mixer after each addition, only until well blended. Stir in the remaining flour mixture from step 1 until well combined and slightly stiff. Cover the dough. Chill for at least 2 hours or overnight.

4. Preheat the oil or shortening (at least 2 inches) in a deep fat fryer or heavy saucepan to 375 degrees on a candy thermometer.
5. Meanwhile, on a lightly rice-floured surface, roll out the dough to a thickness of half an inch. Cut with a 2½-inch rice-floured doughnut cutter. (A biscuit cutter or the rim of a drinking glass can be used as a substitute for a doughnut cutter. Form the doughnut hole by separating a ¾- to 1-inch hole in the center with fingers.)
6. Re-roll dough as necessary. Return warmer dough to chill in the refrigerator while you work with the remaining dough.
7. Fry 3 or 4 doughnuts at a time about one minute on each side, or until golden, turning only once with a slotted spoon. Drain on paper towels.
8. Add desired topping.

Makes 24 doughnuts.

Toppings

Powdered Sugar Doughnuts: Add one cup sifted powdered sugar to a plastic bag. Shake 1-2 doughnuts at a time to coat.

Cinnamon Sugar Doughnuts: Combine one cup sugar and 2½ teaspoons ground cinnamon in a plastic bag. Shake 1-2 doughnuts at a time to coat.

Nutmeg Sugar Doughnuts: Combine one cup sugar and ½ teaspoon ground nutmeg in a plastic bag. Shake doughnuts to coat.

Chocolate Icing: Mix one cup of powdered sugar, two tablespoons unsweetened cocoa powder, and one tablespoon milk or water. Stir in one teaspoon of milk or water at a time until it is of drizzling consistency. Dip the doughnut in the icing and twist to coat.

Lemon Icing: Mix one cup of powdered sugar and one tablespoon of milk or water. Stir in one teaspoon of lemon juice. Stir in one teaspoon milk or water at a time until it is of drizzling consistency. Dip the doughnut in the icing and twist to coat.

Orange Icing: Mix one cup of powdered sugar and one tablespoon of milk or water. Stir in one teaspoon orange juice at a time until it is of drizzling consistency. Dip the doughnut in the icing and twist to coat.

Mocha Icing: Mix one cup of powdered sugar, two tablespoons unsweetened cocoa powder, and one tablespoon liquid coffee, brewed or instant. Stir in one teaspoon of coffee at a time until it is of drizzling consistency. Dip the doughnut in the icing and twist to coat.

Maple Icing: Mix one cup of powdered sugar, ¼ teaspoon vanilla, and one tablespoon of milk or water. Stir in one teaspoon of pure maple syrup at a time until it is of drizzling consistency. Dip the doughnut in the icing and twist to coat.

Pan Toast

Ingredients

½ -1 teaspoon fat (butter, margarine, olive oil, etc.)
2 slices of gluten-free bread

Directions

In a frying pan, add half of your fat of choice. Heat slightly, then add gluten-free bread. Fry until the bread is lightly browned. Lift the bread with a pancake turner and add the remaining amount of fat to the pan. Flip the bread to toast the other side. Fry until lightly browned. Remove from pan and serve hot.

Makes 1 serving.

Note: This toasting technique adds some moisture, as well as a delightful flavor, to the gluten-free breads. It is especially good with the Rice-Tapioca and the Classic White breads in the Bread section, but is also quite tasty with any of the yeast or bread machine breads listed in this book.

Quiche

Ingredients

1 single crust pastry (see page 246)
4 eggs
1½ cups milk or substitute
¼ cup sliced green onions (optional)
¼ teaspoon salt
⅛ teaspoon ground pepper
⅛ teaspoon ground nutmeg
¾ cup cooked, chopped meat (chicken, ham, crabmeat)
    OR ½ cup crumbled bacon
2 cups (about 6 ounces) shredded cheese
    (Swiss, cheddar, Monterey Jack, Havarti)
2 tablespoons sweet rice flour

Directions   *Preheat oven to 325 degrees.*

1. Prepare pastry and follow pre-baking instructions.
2. Meanwhile, in a bowl, combine the eggs, milk, onion (if used), salt, pepper, and nutmeg. Stir in the meat.
3. In another bowl, combine the cheese and the sweet rice flour. Add to the egg mixture.
4. Place the pre-baked, hot piecrust on the center shelf of the preheated oven. Pour the egg mixture into the piecrust.
5. Cook at 325 degrees for 40-45 minutes or until a knife inserted near the center comes out clean.
6. Let stand for 10 minutes before serving.

Makes 6 servings.

Quick Breakfast Rice Pudding

Ingredients

    3 cups milk or substitute
    ½ cup cream of rice cereal
    ¼ cup sugar
    1½ teaspoons vanilla
    Ground nutmeg or ground cinnamon to sprinkle

Directions

1. In a 1½ -quart microwavable casserole, combine milk, cream of rice cereal, sugar, and vanilla.
2. Microwave on high (100%) power for two minutes.
3. Stir, then microwave on high for 30 seconds longer. Repeat until most of the milk has been absorbed.
4. Spoon into individual bowls and sprinkle with ground nutmeg or cinnamon, if desired.

Makes 2 servings.

Variation: For texture more like real rice pudding, stir in 1 cup cooked, chilled rice between steps 3 and 4.

Waffles

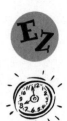

Ingredients

2 cups rice flour
⅓ cup tapioca flour
⅔ cup potato starch flour
3 tablespoons brown sugar
1 tablespoon plus 2 teaspoons baking powder
1½ teaspoons baking soda
¼ teaspoon salt
⅔ cup buttermilk powder
2 beaten eggs
2½ cups milk
2 tablespoons oil

Directions

1. In a bowl, mix the rice flour, tapioca flour, potato starch flour, brown sugar, baking powder, baking soda, salt, and buttermilk powder. Make a well by pressing the ingredients to the sides of the bowl.
2. In a small bowl, mix the eggs, water, and oil.
3. Add the egg mixture to the flour mixture and combine well. Do not over mix. The batter will be slightly lumpy.
4. Drop by ⅓ cupfuls onto a hot waffle iron serving square. Cook according to manufacturer's directions.

Makes 12-14 waffles.

Note: Freeze any extra waffles in a zip-style freezer bag. For a quick breakfast, toast or reheat in the microwave.

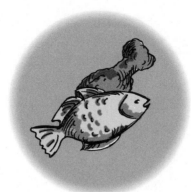

Lunch & Dinner Ideas

Fish ⟁ Meat ⟁ Poultry ⟁ Pizza ⟁ Pasta & Rice

"It's more fun to talk with someone

who doesn't use long, difficult words

but rather short, easy words

like 'What about lunch?'"

—POOH'S LITTLE INSTRUCTION BOOK
inspired by A. A. Milne

"Give a man a fish; you have fed him for today.
Teach a man to fish; and you have fed him for a lifetime."
—Unknown

Fish

Biscuit-Topped Tuna Potpie

Ingredients

1 biscuit recipe (see page 49 or 50, breads)
½ cup chopped onion
¼ cup chopped green pepper
¼ cup chopped celery
¼ cup margarine or butter
¼ cup potato starch flour
¼ cup sweet rice flour
2 teaspoons instant chicken bouillon granules
¼ teaspoon dried thyme, crushed
2½ cups milk
2 cans tuna (6-7 ounces each), drained and flaked
1 tablespoon dried parsley, crushed
1 cup mixed vegetables, cooked

Directions   *Preheat oven to 400 degrees.*

1. Prepare the biscuit dough. Cover and set aside.
2. In a saucepan, cook onion, bell pepper, and celery in butter or margarine until tender.
3. In a small bowl, combine the potato starch flour, sweet rice flour, bouillon, and thyme. Add to the onion mixture and stir until combined.
4. Add the milk all at once. Cook and stir until thickened and bubbly.
5. Stir in tuna, parsley, and mixed vegetables. Cook and stir until heated.
6. Transfer tuna mixture to a two-quart casserole dish. Pat the biscuit dough into patties and cover the casserole completely with the patties. Bake at 400 degrees for 11 to 13 minutes or until the biscuits are lightly browned.

Makes 6 servings.

Hot Tuna Tempties

Ingredients

> 1 can (6-7 ounces) tuna packed in water, drained
> 2 tablespoons chopped green pepper
> 2 tablespoons chopped onion
> 2 tablespoons gluten-free sweet relish
> ½ cup mayonnaise
> 8 slices gluten-free bread
> 4 slices American cheese (about 4 ounces)

Directions

Preheat oven to 350 degrees.

1. Combine the tuna, green pepper, onion, sweet relish, and mayonnaise in a small bowl.
2. Tear off four squares of foil. Put one slice of bread on each piece of foil. Top each bread slice with ¼ of the tuna mixture and one slice of the American cheese. Top with the remaining bread slices.
3. Wrap the foil around each sandwich and bake in a 350-degree oven for 14-15 minutes or until heated through.

Makes 4 sandwiches.

Variation: Use canned chicken or turkey instead of tuna.

Pan Fried Fish

Ingredients

2 pounds fresh or frozen fish filets (½ to 1 inch thick)
2 beaten eggs
¼ cup water
1 cup corn meal
⅓ cup potato starch flour
1 teaspoon salt
¼ teaspoon pepper
Oil for frying (corn, canola, vegetable, olive, etc.)

Directions

1. Thaw fish, if frozen. Cut fish into serving size portions. Pat dry with paper towels.
2. In a shallow dish or pie pan, combine eggs and water.
3. In a zip-style bag, mix corn meal, potato starch flour, salt, and pepper. (Or mix in another shallow dish.)
4. Preheat 1 inch of oil in a heavy frying pan until 375 degrees on a candy thermometer or until a droplet of water crackles when added to the oil.
5. Dip the fish in the egg mixture then coat with the flour mixture.
6. Fry fish in hot oil on one side until golden (3-4 minutes for ½-inch thickness, 5-6 minutes for 1-inch thickness). Turn carefully. Fry other side until golden and fish flakes easily with a fork.
7. Drain on paper towels. Keep warm in a 200-degree oven while frying remaining fish.

Makes 6-8 servings.

Salmon Patties

Ingredients

2 cans (6 ounces each) skinless boneless salmon, drained
½ cup plain rice or corn cakes, crushed (or gluten-free crackers)
1 egg, beaten
Oil for cooking

Directions

1. Place the salmon, rice cake crumbs, and beaten egg in a bowl. Combine well.
2. Pour just enough oil (1-2 tablespoons) to lightly coat a medium-sized frying pan. Heat oil until it crackles when water droplets are sprinkled on it.
3. Divide fish mixture into fourths. Form each portion into a patty.
4. Fry the patties in the hot oil for 3-4 minutes or until golden on the bottom. Flip the patties carefully and fry the other side until golden and crispy. (NOTE: Only turn the fish once to prevent the patty from falling apart.)
5. Serve immediately. This recipe does not reheat well.

Makes 4 servings.

Serving suggestion: Serve with macaroni and cheese and a salad.

Tuna Casserole

Ingredients

2¼ cups (8 oz.) gluten-free macaroni
2 tablespoons margarine or butter
1 teaspoon minced garlic (two cloves)
½ teaspoon dried basil, crushed
2 tablespoons potato starch flour or cornstarch
1½ cup milk or substitute
½ cup grated Parmesan cheese (2 ounces)
1 can (6-7 ounces) light tuna in water, drained
½ cup fresh or frozen sweet peas (optional)
1 slice gluten-free toast, crumbled (⅓ cup)

Directions

Preheat oven to 400 degrees.

1. In a large saucepan, prepare macaroni according to package directions. Drain well in a colander and rinse with hot water. Set colander with noodles aside.
2. Melt the margarine in the saucepan. Add the garlic, basil, and potato starch flour and stir until margarine is absorbed.
3. Add the milk all at once. Cook until thickened and bubbly. Cook one minute more. Remove from heat.
4. Add the Parmesan cheese, tuna, cooked macaroni, and peas, if used, to the white sauce. Stir gently to combine.
5. Pour into a 2-quart casserole dish. Top with toasted breadcrumbs.
6. Bake in a 400-degree oven for 20 to 25 minutes or until mixture is bubbly and breadcrumbs are browned.

Makes 6-8 servings.

"There's no such thing as a tough child—
if you parboil them first for seven hours they always come out tender."
—W. C. Fields

Meats

Arroz con Puerco

▪▪▪▪▪▪▪▪▪▪▪▪▪▪▪▪▪▪▪▪▪

A Spanish term meaning rice and pork.

Ingredients

4 pork loin chops (about 1½ pounds)
1 tablespoon oil
2 14½-ounce cans tomatoes, cut up
1 cup frozen corn (optional)
½ cup long grain rice
½ cup diced green chilies (4-ounce can)
½ teaspoon chili powder
½ teaspoon basil, crushed
¼ teaspoon oregano, crushed
½ teaspoon onion powder (optional)
1 15-ounce can garbanzo beans or kidney beans, drained
Corn tortillas or Mock Flour Tortillas (page 53)

Directions   *Preheat oven to 350 degrees.*

1. In a skillet, brown chops in oil for five minutes a side.
2. Remove the chops from the pan and drain on paper towels. Drain the fat from pan.
3. Combine undrained tomatoes, corn (if used), rice, undrained green chilies, chili powder, basil, oregano, and onion powder (if used) in the same skillet used to cook the chops. Heat to boiling. Add the beans, and boil for one minute.
4. Transfer the vegetable mixture into a 3- to 4-quart casserole dish. Arrange chops on top and sprinkle with salt and pepper, if desired.
5. Cover and bake for 30 minutes. Remove cover and bake 10 to 12 minutes or until the rice is tender and the chops are no longer pink.
6. Meanwhile, wrap tortillas in foil and heat with the casserole for the last 5 to 8 minutes or until hot.
7. Serve the casserole with hot tortillas.

Makes 4 main dish servings.

Serving suggestion: Wrap the rice in tortillas and eat like burritos with chops on the side. Or cut the chops into strips, wrap the meat and rice mixture in the tortillas, and eat like fajitas.

Barbecue Sauce

Use this sweet and tangy sauce as a substitute for barbecue sauce in any recipe.

Ingredients

½ cup ketchup (4 ounces)
1 6-ounce can tomato paste
¼ cup red wine or apple cider vinegar
2 tablespoons sugar
1 tablespoon gluten-free Worcestershire sauce
1 tablespoon prepared yellow mustard
½ teaspoon celery seed
½ cup water
¼ teaspoon salt

Directions

1. Combine all ingredients in a 2-quart saucepan.
2. Bring to a boil. Reduce heat and simmer 10-15 minutes or to desired consistency.

Makes 1¾ cups.

Honey Barbecue Sauce: Prepare as above except add ¼ cup honey before boiling.

Bell Pepper Boats

Ingredients

½ pound ground beef or turkey
½ pound ground sausage
4 large green bell peppers
½ cup diced green chilies, drained (4-ounce can) *(optional)*
1 14½-ounce can tomatoes, cut up
1 15-ounce can tomato sauce
1 teaspoon oregano
½ teaspoon cumin *(optional)*
1 cup water
1 cup rice, uncooked
1 cup shredded cheddar cheese
3-4 large stalks celery
4 thick slices of cheddar cheese

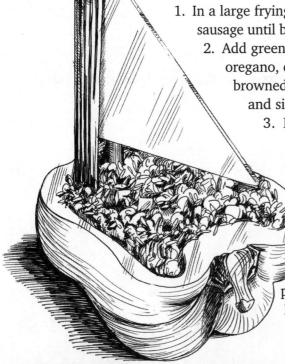

Directions

1. In a large frying pan, cook ground beef or turkey and sausage until brown. Drain the meats and return to the pan.
2. Add green chilies (if used), tomatoes, tomato sauce, oregano, cumin (if used), water, and the rice to the browned meat. Bring to a boil. Reduce heat, cover, and simmer for 20 minutes. Stir occasionally.
3. Meanwhile, put on a small pan of water to boil. Cut the bell peppers in half, through the stem to the bottom. Remove the seeds and rinse well. Boil each pepper half for 1½ minutes. Drain on paper towels. Set aside.
4. Preheat oven to 375 degrees.
5. Add the shredded cheese to the rice mixture and stir until melted. Spoon into pepper halves. Place in a shallow baking dish. Bake in a 375-degree oven for 15 minutes.

6. Meanwhile prepare the "masts" by washing the celery stalks in cold water. Cut the celery stalks into 4-inch lengths. Cut the cheese slices diagonally into 8 triangle "sails." Set aside.

7. Remove baked peppers from the oven. Turn oven off.

8. Slide the longest side of a cheese "sail" into the hollow section of a celery stick. Stuff your "mast" and "sail" combination into one end of the baked pepper "boat," pressing the bottom edge of the "sail" into the rice mixture. Repeat with remaining boats. (See illustration)

Makes 8 individual boat servings.

Cheesy Hamburger Casserole
■■■■■■■■■■■■■■■■■■■■■■■■

Ingredients

3 cups gluten-free macaroni or Rotini noodles
½ pound ground hamburger or turkey
½ cup chopped onion (1 medium)
½ medium bell pepper, chopped
2 cloves garlic, minced
1 tablespoon dried parsley, crushed
1½ teaspoons dried basil, crushed
1 14½-ounce can tomatoes, cut up
1½ cups shredded cheddar cheese (6 ounces)
1 cup shredded mozzarella cheese (4 ounces)
½ cup milk
1 teaspoon ground pepper *(optional)*
1 tablespoon sweet rice flour or white rice flour
½ cup grated Parmesan cheese (2 ounces) or gluten-free breadcrumbs

Directions   *Preheat oven to 350 degrees.*

1. In a large saucepan, cook the noodles according to package directions. Drain. Return drained noodles to pan.
2. Meanwhile, in a skillet sauté the hamburger or turkey, onion, bell pepper, and garlic. Add the parsley, basil, tomatoes, cheddar cheese, mozzarella cheese, milk, ground pepper (if used), and sweet rice flour. Mix well. Remove from heat.
3. Add the hamburger mixture to the drained noodles. Stir to combine.
4. Transfer to a 1½-quart casserole dish. Sprinkle with the Parmesan cheese or breadcrumbs.
5. Bake in a 350-degree oven for 20 minutes or until heated through and edges are browned.

Makes 8 servings.

Note: The vegetables listed are optional; the flavor and consistency may change with the substitute you choose.

Corn Dogs

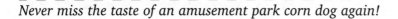

Never miss the taste of an amusement park corn dog again!

Ingredients

8-10 gluten-free hot dogs (1 pound)
½ cup rice flour
¼ cup tapioca flour
¼ cup potato starch flour
⅔ cup corn meal
2 tablespoons sugar
1½ teaspoons baking powder
½ teaspoon dry mustard
1 beaten egg
¾ cup milk or substitute
2 tablespoons cooking oil
Extra rice flour
Shortening *or* cooking oil for deep-fat frying

Directions

1. Pat hot dogs dry with paper towels. If desired, insert a wooden skewer into one end of each hot dog. Set aside.
2. In a shallow bowl or pie pan, combine the rice flour, tapioca flour, potato starch flour, corn meal, sugar, baking powder, and dry mustard.
3. In another bowl, combine the beaten egg, milk, and the 2 tablespoons of oil. Add to the dry ingredients and mix well. The batter will be thick.
4. Measure ¾-inch of shortening or oil into a deep frying pan. Heat until a candy thermometer reads 375 degrees. (Or use a deep fat fryer according to the manufacturer's directions.)
5. Put some extra rice flour on a shallow plate. Roll the hot dogs in the additional rice flour. (This prevents the cornbread coating from falling off the hot dog during frying.) Then coat the hot dogs with the batter.

6. Fry the hot dogs, three at a time, turning with tongs after 10 seconds. Cook for about 1 minute more, or until golden brown; turn and cook for about 1 minute more. Drain on paper towels.

7. Keep warm in a slightly warmed oven (200 degrees) or inside the microwave without turning it on.

Makes 8-10 corn dogs.

Serving Suggestion: Serve corndogs with gluten-free ketchup or mustard, if desired, and Baked Garlic Parmesan Fries (see page 183).

Kielbasa and Rice

Ingredients

1 pound kielbasa or polish sausage, cut into bite-sized pieces
1 cup Chinese style pea pods (8 ounces)
1 tablespoon potato starch flour
2 cups milk or substitute (16 ounces)
1 cup grated Parmesan cheese (4 ounces)
6 cups hot cooked rice (2 cups uncooked)

Directions

1. In a large skillet, fry the kielbasa until brown. Remove from skillet and drain on paper towels, reserving the pan drippings.
2. In the skillet, heat the pea pods and pan drippings for three minutes. Push the pea pods to the sides of the skillet.
3. Stir the potato starch flour into the drippings.
4. Add the milk all at once. Cook and stir until slightly thickened and bubbly.
5. Add the Parmesan cheese and cook one minute more.
6. Return the sausages to the skillet and heat through.

Makes 6 servings.

Serving Suggestion: Serve over the hot rice.

Lasagna

■▲■▲■▲■■▲■▲■■▲■■■▲■■■■▲■■■

A tasty and easy lasagna, beginning with dry rice or corn lasagna noodles. It whips up fairly quick and is a cheesy treat!

Ingredients

¾ pound ground beef or turkey
1 cup chopped onion (1 medium)
2 cloves garlic, minced
1 15-ounce can tomato sauce
2 teaspoons crushed dried basil
1 teaspoon crushed, dried oregano
1 cup sliced (or chopped) black olives (8 ounces) *(optional)*
10 ounces gluten-free lasagna noodles (about 10)
1 beaten egg
2 cups ricotta or cottage cheese (16 ounces)
1 cup grated Parmesan cheese (4 ounces)
1 tablespoon dried parsley flakes
6 cups shredded mozzarella cheese (24 ounces)

Directions   *Preheat oven to 375 degrees.*

1. In a large saucepan, cook the meat, onion, and garlic until the meat is brown and the onion is tender. Drain any fat.
2. Stir in tomato sauce, basil, oregano, and ½ cup of the olives (if used). Bring to boiling; reduce heat. Cover and simmer for 15 minutes, stirring occasionally.
3. Meanwhile, lightly coat the bottom of a 13 x 9 x 2-inch baking dish with non-stick cooking spray or oil.
4. For filling, in a separate mixing bowl, combine the egg, ricotta or cottage cheese, ¾ cup of the Parmesan cheese, and the parsley flakes by beating with an electric mixer until smooth (or process in a food processor).
5. Layer half of the uncooked noodles in the prepared baking dish. Spread with half of the meat sauce. Spread half of the egg and cheese

filling over the meat sauce. Top with half of the mozzarella cheese. Repeat the layers. Top with the remaining olives (if used) and then sprinkle the remaining ¼ cup Parmesan cheese on top.

6. Cover the dish with foil and bake in a 375-degree oven for 35 minutes.
7. Uncover and bake an additional 20 minutes or until heated through and the noodles are tender. Let stand 10 minutes before slicing.

Makes 8 servings.

Serving suggestion: Serve with Garlic Toast (page 64) or Garlic Biscuits (page 52) and a tossed green salad.

Meaty Beef Meatloaf

If your family leaves a morsel behind, you may be able to make a great meatloaf sandwich with the cooled leftovers. Or make a second loaf just for sandwiches.

Ingredients

1 large egg, beaten
1 cup celery, chopped (2 stalks)
¼ cup onion, chopped (*optional*)
½ teaspoon dried basil or dill weed
½ teaspoon salt
½ teaspoon pepper
¾ cup tomato paste (1 6-ounce can)
1 teaspoon Worcestershire sauce or A-1® steak sauce (*optional*)
½ cup gluten-free cracker crumbs (3½ ounces) OR 1 cup gluten-free
    bread crumbs (1-2 slices)
1 pound lean ground beef

Directions   *Preheat oven to 350 degrees.*

1. In a large bowl, combine the egg, celery, onion, basil or dill weed, salt, pepper, tomato paste, and Worcestershire sauce or A-1® steak sauce, if used.
2. Add the cracker crumbs or crumbled bread and toss to coat.
3. Add the ground beef and mix well.
4. Transfer into a 1½-quart casserole or large loaf pan. Bake, uncovered, in a 350-degree oven for 50 minutes.
5. Remove the meatloaf from the oven. Spoon off any excess fat and discard.
6. Return the meatloaf to the oven and heat an additional 5-10 minutes or until no longer pink and internal temperature on a meat thermometer is 170 degrees.
7. Serve with ketchup or steak sauce, if desired.

Makes 6 servings.

Serving suggestion: Serve with mashed potatoes, Green Bean Amandine (recipe page 189), and warm gluten-free bread.

Meatloaf Patties: Prepare as above through step 3, and then form into 6 patties. Fry in a lightly oiled pan for 5-10 minutes, turning once or until no longer pink and internal temperature on a meat thermometer is 170 degrees.

One Skillet Beef Stroganoff

Ingredients

1 pound ground beef or turkey

1 clove garlic, minced

¼ cup chopped onion

3 teaspoons beef bouillon granules (3 cubes)

8 ounces gluten-free lasagna noodles (about 8),
    broken into one-inch pieces

1 cup sour cream (about 8 ounces)

2 tablespoons rice flour

¼ teaspoon pepper

Directions

1. In a large skillet with a lid, sauté meat with garlic and onion over medium heat until the meat is brown and the onion is tender and translucent.
2. Add 5 cups of water and bouillon to the skillet. Bring to a boil.
3. Add the lasagna noodles. Return to a boil. Reduce heat and cover. Cook for 15 to 20 minutes or until the noodles are tender and water is absorbed. (Note: add more water if needed, ½ cup at a time.)
4. Meanwhile, combine the sour cream, rice flour, 2 tablespoons of water, and pepper in a small bowl. Set aside.
5. When the noodles are done, add the sour cream mixture to the skillet. Cook and stir over medium heat until bubbly. Cook and stir one minute more.

Makes 4 servings.

Serving suggestion: Serve with applesauce, Green Beans almandine (page 89), and Mock Rye Bread (page 67.)

Porcupine Meatballs

Ingredients

1 beaten egg
¾ cup V-8® juice (12-ounce can) or a 10¾-ounce can
  of gluten-free tomato soup or ¾ cup tomato soup (page 196)
¼ cup long grain rice, uncooked
¼ teaspoon onion powder
¼ teaspoon pepper
1 pound ground beef or turkey
1 teaspoon gluten-free steak sauce (such as A-1®)
½ teaspoon dried, crushed oregano

Directions

1. In a medium-sized bowl, combine the egg, ¼ cup of the V-8® juice, the uncooked rice, onion powder, and pepper. Add the ground meat and mix well.
2. Shape into 20 meatballs. Place in a large skillet.
3. In a small bowl, mix remaining V-8® juice with the steak sauce, oregano, and ½ cup of water. Pour over the meatballs.
4. Bring the meatball mixture to a boil, then reduce heat. Cover and simmer, stirring often for 20 minutes or until no pink remains and the rice is tender.
5. Skim the fat. Serve with Parmesan cheese, if desired.

Makes 4 servings.

Pork Chops with Herb Gravy

Ingredients

4 pork chops, cut ¾-inch thick
2 tablespoons margarine or butter
1 medium carrot, peeled and shredded
1 teaspoon dried parsley, crushed
1 tablespoon sweet rice flour
½ teaspoon dried basil, crushed
½ teaspoon beef bouillon granules
¼ teaspoon pepper
⅔ cup milk or milk substitute

Directions

1. Trim the fat from the chops. In a large skillet, cook the chops in the margarine over medium heat for five minutes.
2. Turn the chops and add carrot. Cook for five to seven minutes more or until no pink remains. Remove the chops from the pan and set aside.
3. In the same skillet, stir parsley, sweet rice flour, bouillon granules, and pepper into the drippings and carrots.
4. Cook for 30 seconds, then add the milk all at once. Cook and stir the gravy until thickened and bubbly.
5. Return the chops to the pan and heat through.
6. Serve the chops with the gravy spooned on top.

Makes 4 servings.

Pot Roast

▪▪▪▪▪▪▪▪▪▪▪▪▪▪▪▪▪▪▪▪▪▪▪

Ingredients

½ cup rice flour
⅛ teaspoon pepper
⅛ teaspoon salt
3-4 pound beef chuck pot roast or pork loin roast
2 tablespoons vegetable oil
2 teaspoons beef bouillon granules (or 2 cubes)
1 large bay leaf
1½ teaspoons basil
¾ teaspoon oregano
4-5 medium potatoes, cut into eighths or 15-20 new potatoes, halved
3-4 large carrots, cut into 1-inch pieces
1 large onion, cut into eighths
3-4 celery stalks, cut into 1-inch pieces
Up to ¼ cup potato starch flour

Directions

1. Place rice flour, pepper, and salt in a large zip-style bag. Shake to combine. Add the roast. Shake to coat.
2. In a large Dutch oven, brown the roast in hot oil on all sides. (Reserve remaining flour mixture for gravy.)
3. Add bouillon granules, bay leaf, basil, and oregano to Dutch oven. Add 1½ cups of water.
4. Bring to a boil. Cover, reduce heat, and simmer for 1¼ hours.
5. Add potatoes, carrots, onion, and celery. Return to a boil. Cover, reduce heat, and simmer for an additional 25-30 minutes or until the meat and vegetables are tender.
6. Remove meat and vegetables from the pan. Discard the bay leaf.
7. For the gravy, skim the fat from the pan juices and discard. Measure 1½ cups of the juices. (Discard the remaining juices or save for use later, such as a soup base.) Return the measured juices to the pan. Heat to gentle boil.

8. Pour the leftover flour mixture into a measuring cup, adding enough potato starch flour to make ¼ cup total. Combine the flour with ½ cup of cold water. Mix well until no lumps are seen. Add to the pan, stirring constantly. Cook and stir until thickened and bubbly. Cook for one minute longer.
9. Pass the gravy with the meat.

Makes 8 servings.

Serving Suggestion: Serve with warm Classic White bread (recipe page 62) or Buttermilk Biscuits (recipe page 50).

Sausage Topped Macaroni Casserole

Ingredients

8 ounces gluten-free macaroni (makes 4 cups, cooked)

¾ cup V-8® juice (12-ounce can) or a 10¾-ounce can of gluten-free tomato soup or ¾ cup tomato soup (page 196)

1 tablespoon potato starch flour or cornstarch

¼ cup onion, chopped

¼ cup green bell pepper, chopped

1 teaspoon salt

¼ teaspoon pepper

8 gluten-free sausage links

½ cup shredded cheddar cheese (2 ounces)

Directions   *Preheat oven to 350 degrees.*

1. Cook macaroni in boiling water until tender. Drain and rinse with hot water. Set aside.
2. In the same pan, combine V-8® juice, potato starch, onion, bell pepper, salt, pepper, and ½ cup of water. Simmer for 10 minutes over low heat.
3. In a skillet, brown the sausage links on all sides, about 5 minutes.
4. Fold the macaroni and the cheese into the V-8® mixture.
5. Pour the macaroni mixture into a well-buttered or greased 1½-quart casserole dish. Arrange the sausages over the macaroni mixture.
6. Bake in a 350-degree oven for 45-50 minutes or until the sausages are thoroughly cooked and the mixture is hot and bubbly.

Makes 4 servings.

Sloppy Joes

Ingredients

1 pound ground beef or turkey

¼ cup chopped onion

¼ cup chopped green pepper

1 clove garlic, minced

1 4-ounce can tomato paste

1 tablespoon vinegar

1 tablespoon sugar

1 teaspoon salt

½ teaspoon chili powder

¼ teaspoon cumin

¼ teaspoon oregano

¼ teaspoon ground coriander

¼ teaspoon xanthan gum

6 gluten-free hamburger buns (see page 65)

Directions

1. In a large skillet, sauté the ground beef or turkey, onion, green pepper, and garlic until the meat is browned and the onions are translucent.
2. Add tomato paste, vinegar, sugar, salt, chili powder, cumin, oregano, coriander, xanthan gum, and ½ cup of water. Heat to boiling, then reduce heat and simmer for 10 minutes.
3. Meanwhile, toast the hamburger buns, if desired.
4. Spoon the meat mixture onto the bottom halves of the buns. Add the tops of the buns.

Makes 6 sandwiches.

Serving suggestion: Serve with Baked Garlic Parmesan Fries (page 183), hot French fries, or your favorite chips.

Spaghetti Pie

Ingredients

4 ounces rice or corn spaghetti
½ pound ground beef, turkey, sausage, or combination
½ cup chopped onion *(optional)*
½ cup chopped green pepper (½ medium)
¾ cup spaghetti or pizza sauce (15 ounces)
2 eggs
⅓ cup grated Parmesan cheese (1⅓ ounces)
1 tablespoon butter or margarine, melted
1 cup cottage cheese (8 ounces)
½ cup shredded mozzarella cheese (2 ounces)

Directions   *Preheat oven to 350 degrees.*

1. Cook spaghetti according to package directions. Drain well. Return to pan.
2. Meanwhile, in a frying pan, sauté the ground meat, onions, and green pepper until the meat is browned and the onions are translucent. Drain fats. Add spaghetti or pizza sauce and stir to combine. Set aside.
3. In a bowl, beat one egg. Add the Parmesan cheese and melted butter, and mix well to combine. Add to the hot pasta and toss until combined.
4. In a well-greased 9-inch pie pan, spread the spaghetti mixture with a spoon (or cover the mixture with plastic wrap and smooth with hands, then remove plastic wrap) across the bottom and up the sides to form a crust.
5. Beat the remaining egg in a small bowl. Drain the cottage cheese, then combine with beaten egg. Spread over the bottom of the crust.
6. Spoon the meat mixture over the cottage cheese mixture.
7. Bake in a 350-degree oven for 20 minutes. Remove from oven.
8. Sprinkle mozzarella cheese over the top of the pie. Return the pie to the oven for 5-8 minutes more or until the cheese melts and the crust sets. Let stand for 5 minutes before slicing into wedges.

Makes 6 servings.

Spanish Rice Wraps

Ingredients

1 pound ground turkey or beef
1 clove garlic, minced
½ cup chopped green pepper (½ medium)
1 14½-ounce can tomatoes, chopped
1 15-ounce can tomato sauce
1 cup rice
1 dozen corn tortillas or Mock Flour Tortillas (page 53)
1½ cups shredded cheddar cheese (about 12 ounces)

Directions

1. In a large skillet, sauté meat with the garlic and green pepper. (If using beef, drain, then return to skillet.)
2. Add tomatoes, tomato sauce, and 1 cup of water to the meat. Bring to a boil.
3. Add the rice to the skillet, cover, and reduce heat. Simmer for 20 minutes or until rice is tender.
4. Meanwhile, wrap the tortillas in foil and heat in a 350-degree oven for 10 minutes or until soft. (Or microwave in a moist towel until soft.)
5. Lay tortillas on a flat surface. Spoon rice mixture on one-half of each tortilla. Top with ¼ cup of the shredded cheese. Fold the other half of the tortilla over, taco style.

Microwave Directions

Follow steps 1 through 3. Pour into a microwave-safe casserole dish and cover. Heat on high for 20 minutes or until the rice is tender. Continue with steps 4 and 5 above.

Makes 6 servings.

Serving suggestion: Serve with corn chips and salsa.

Soft Tacos

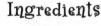

Ingredients

1 pound ground turkey or beef
½ cup chopped onion (1 small)
½ cup diced green chilies, drained (4-ounce can)
1–1½ teaspoons chili powder
12 corn tortillas or Mock Flour tortillas (page 53)
2 cups shredded cheddar cheese

Toppings

1½ cups shredded lettuce
1 cup diced tomatoes (1 large)
½ cup sour cream (4 ounces)
½ cup sliced black olives, drained (4-ounce can)

Directions

1. Sauté the ground turkey or beef and onions. (If using beef, drain the fat.) Add the green chilies and the chili powder to taste. Stir to combine, then remove from heat.
2. On an ungreased hot griddle or frying pan, heat tortillas for 1 minute.
3. Spoon meat mixture onto ½ of a tortilla. Top with shredded cheddar cheese. Fold in half and heat for about 20 seconds more. Turn the taco over and heat until the cheese melts, about 20 seconds on stovetop. Remove from heat.
4. Top with lettuce, tomatoes, sour cream (if used), and black olives (if used).

Makes 12 soft tacos.

Tacos

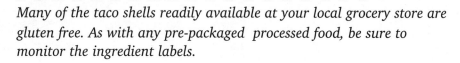

Many of the taco shells readily available at your local grocery store are gluten free. As with any pre-packaged processed food, be sure to monitor the ingredient labels.

Ingredients

12 gluten-free taco shells
1 pound ground turkey or beef
½ cup chopped onion
½ cup diced green chilies, drained (4-ounce can)
1–1½ teaspoons chili powder

Toppings

1 cup shredded cheddar cheese
1½ cups shredded lettuce
1 cup diced tomatoes
½ cup sour cream *(optional)*
½ cup sliced black olives, drained (4-ounce can) *(optional)*

Directions   ***Preheat oven to 350 degrees.***

1. Sauté the ground turkey or beef and onions. (If using beef, drain the fat.) Add the green chilies and the chili powder, to taste. Stir to combine. Heat for 1 minute, then remove from heat.
2. Meanwhile, heat the taco shells in 350-degree oven for 5 minutes. Remove from oven.
3. Spoon meat mixture into taco shells. Top with shredded cheddar cheese, lettuce, tomatoes, sour cream (if used), and black olives (if used).

Makes 12 tacos.

"If parents pass enthusiasm along to their children,
they will have left them an estate of incalculable value."
—Thomas Edison

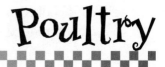

Chicken Biscuit Surprise

Ingredients

1 Buttermilk Biscuit recipe (page 50)
2 cups cooked shredded chicken (or 2 12½-ounce cans, drained)
2 cups shredded cheddar or Swiss cheese (about ½ pound)

Directions

Preheat oven to 450 degrees.

1. Place one heaping tablespoon of the biscuit dough in the bottoms of each of 18 well-greased muffin cups. Drop 2 tablespoons of shredded chicken on each biscuit. Layer each biscuit with 2 tablespoons of the cheese. Cover each biscuit with another heaping tablespoon of biscuit dough.
2. Bake at 450 degrees for 15-17 minutes or until a toothpick inserted near the center of the biscuit comes out clean and the biscuits are golden.
3. Invert onto a cooling rack and serve immediately.

Makes 9 two-sandwich servings.

Chicken Nuggets

Ingredients

3 tablespoons margarine or butter, melted

2 teaspoons gluten-free Worcestershire sauce

2 whole, large chicken breasts, skinned, boned, and cut into 1-inch pieces (or about 15 chicken tenderloins cut into fourths) (about 1½ pounds)

1 cup plain potato chips or gluten-free corn flakes, crushed to about ½ cup

¼ cup grated Parmesan cheese (1 ounce)

Directions

Preheat oven to 450 degrees.

1. Stir together margarine and Worcestershire sauce in a small, flat bowl or pie pan. Add a few pieces of the chicken to coat.
2. In a plastic bag, combine the crushed chips and the Parmesan cheese. Add the margarine-coated pieces of chicken and shake well. Place the pieces in a single layer on a lightly greased cookie sheet with a ½-inch lip or on a shallow baking dish. Repeat with the remaining chicken pieces.
3. Bake in a preheated 450-degree oven for 9-10 minutes, or until the chicken is no longer pink inside.

Makes 3-4 servings.

Barbecue Chicken Nuggets: Prepare as above, substituting barbecue-flavored potato chips for the plain chips or corn flakes.

Chicken with Dijon Sauce

Ingredients

1 cup long grain rice, uncooked

8 boneless, skinless chicken tenderloins
  (or 4 breasts, cut in half lengthwise)

2-3 teaspoons lemon-pepper seasoning

½-1 teaspoon onion powder *(optional)*

¼ cup margarine or butter

2 tablespoons rice, potato starch, or arrowroot flour

2 cups light cream or milk

2 tablespoons gluten-free Dijon-style mustard

Directions

Preheat oven to 350 degrees.

1. In a saucepan, bring the long grain rice and 2 cups water to a boil. Cover and reduce heat. Cook rice for 20 minutes or until rice is tender and water is absorbed.

2. Meanwhile, rinse chicken in water and pat dry. Sprinkle lemon-pepper seasoning and onion powder, if used, over the chicken.

3. In a frying pan, melt the margarine. Add seasoned chicken. Cook until juices run clear and no pink remains, turning once or twice. Remove chicken from pan, set aside, and keep warm.

4. Add the rice flour to the frying pan. Cook for 15 seconds. Add the light cream or milk all at once. Cook and stir until thick and bubbly, stirring constantly. Cook one minute more. Add the Dijon mustard and stir to combine. Remove from heat.

5. Serve chicken over a bed of rice and top with the Dijon gravy.

Makes 4 servings.

Serving suggestion: Serve with tomatos wedges and carrot and celery sticks, if desired.

Deep Fried Chicken Nuggets

Ingredients

15 chicken tenderloins or 2 whole skinless, boneless
  chicken breasts, cut into 1-inch squares (about 1½ pounds)
¼ cup plus 2 tablespoons rice flour
¼ cup potato starch flour
2 tablespoons tapioca flour
¼ cup corn meal
½ teaspoon sugar
½ teaspoon salt
Dash of pepper (to taste)
1 beaten egg
2 tablespoons cooking oil
½ cup cold water
Oil for frying

Directions

Preheat oven to 350 degrees.

1. Pour 1½-2 inches of oil into a heavy 3-quart saucepan or deep fat fryer. Heat oil to 365 degrees on a candy thermometer.
2. Meanwhile, rinse the chicken pieces well and pat dry in a cotton (or lint-free) tea towel.
3. In a bowl, combine the rice flour, potato starch flour, tapioca flour, corn meal, sugar, salt, and pepper. Make a well in the center.
4. In another bowl, combine the beaten egg, the 2 tablespoons of oil, and ¼ cup of the water. Add to the flour mixture. Combine well and add the rest of the water a tablespoon at a time until a thick, yet smooth batter forms.
5. Dip 5-6 pieces of the dried chicken pieces into the batter, coating well. Carefully drop the battered chicken into the hot oil. Cook for about a minute or until golden brown.
6. Turn the nuggets and cook another minute until golden brown and the chicken is no longer pink.
7. Remove the nuggets from the hot oil with a slotted spoon. Drain on a plate covered with paper toweling.
8. Repeat steps 5-7 with remaining chicken pieces.
9. Serve immediately or keep warm in a 200-degree oven in an ovenproof dish.

Makes 3-4 servings.

Dilled Chicken & Rice Casserole

Ingredients

1 cup rice, uncooked
1 cup chopped celery (2 stalks)
½ cup chopped onion (1 medium)
¼ cup chopped green bell pepper (¼ medium)
3 tablespoons margarine or butter
3 tablespoons potato starch flour
1½ teaspoons salt
⅛ teaspoon pepper (if desired)
1¾ cups milk
1 tablespoon dried parsley, crushed
1-3 teaspoons dried dill weed, crushed (to taste)
1 cup sour cream (or non-dairy sour cream substitute)
2 cups cubed cooked chicken (or turkey)
½ cup toasted, crushed gluten-free bread crumbs (see note below)

Directions

Preheat oven to 350 degrees.

1. Cook rice according to package directions.
2. Meanwhile, in a large saucepan, cook the celery, onion, and bell pepper in the margarine until tender and onions are translucent.
3. Stir in the potato starch flour, salt, and pepper (if used).
4. Add the milk all at once, stirring constantly until thickened and bubbly. Cook for 2 minutes more.
5. Stir in parsley and dill. Remove the pan from the heat and stir in the sour cream.
6. Stir in the rice and chicken.
7. Pour into a 1½-quart casserole dish. Top with the breadcrumbs.
8. Bake, uncovered, at 350 degrees for 35 to 40 minutes, or until heated.

Makes 6 servings.

Note: To make the bread crumbs, toast day-old bread slices. Crumble the toasted pieces with your fingers or chop in a food processor to the desired size.

Dilled Chicken Noodle Casserole: Prepare as above, but substitute 2 cups of cooked gluten-free noodles for the rice.

Green Chili Casserole

This casserole is like a layered enchilada. It freezes well and actually tastes even better the second day!

Ingredients

2 skinless, boneless chicken breasts, cooked and cubed (about 2 cups)
1 recipe cream of chicken soup (4½ cups) (page 196)
½ cup diced green chilies (4-ounce can)
½ cup chopped onion *(optional)*
5 cups shredded mild cheddar cheese (1¼ pound)
18 corn tortillas

Directions   ***Preheat oven to 350 degrees.***

1. In a large saucepan, heat cubed chicken, chicken soup, chilies, and onion, if used, to a boil. Remove from heat.
2. In a large, shallow casserole, lay six tortillas flat. Pour one third of the chicken mixture over the tortillas and cover with one third of the cheese. Repeat layers two times.
3. Bake, uncovered, at 350 degrees for 45 minutes or until mixture bubbles and cheese is melted.

Makes 6-8 servings.

Serving suggestion: Serve with tossed green salad and tortilla chips.

Spanish Chicken & Rice

Ingredients

2 whole skinless, boneless chicken breasts (1½ pounds)
2 tablespoons oil
½ cup chopped green pepper
½ cup chopped celery
½ cup chopped onion *(optional)*
1 clove garlic, minced
3½ cups tomatoes, diced (2 14½-ounce cans)
¾ cup long grain rice, uncooked
1½ teaspoons chili powder
1 teaspoon sugar
1 cup shredded cheddar cheese (4 ounces)

Directions

1. In a large skillet with a lid, cook the chicken in one tablespoon of the oil. Remove from pan and set aside.
2. Add remaining oil, green pepper, celery, onion (if used), and garlic to the skillet. Cook over low heat until vegetables are tender, but not yet browned.
3. Meanwhile, cube the chicken breasts and add to the pan. Stir in undrained tomatoes, rice, chili powder, sugar, and one cup of water. Bring to a boil.
4. Reduce heat, cover, and simmer for 20 minutes or until the rice is tender and most of the liquid is absorbed. Remove from heat.
5. Sprinkle with the cheddar cheese. Cover and let stand for five minutes or until cheese melts.

Makes 6 servings.

Serving suggestion: Serve with warm tortillas or bread and a salad.

Ground Turkey Meatloaf EZ

Ingredients

1 large egg, beaten
1 cup celery, chopped (2 stalks)
¼ cup onion, chopped (½ medium)
½ teaspoon poultry seasoning
½ teaspoon salt
½ teaspoon pepper
¾ cup tomato paste (6-ounce can)
1 teaspoon Worcestershire sauce *(optional)*
½ cup gluten-free cracker crumbs (3½ ounces) OR 1 cup gluten-free
   bread crumbs (1-2 slices)
1 pound ground turkey

Directions   *Preheat oven to 350 degrees.*

1. In a large bowl, combine the egg, celery, onion, poultry seasoning,
   salt, pepper, tomato paste, and Worcestershire sauce, if used.
2. Add the cracker or bread crumbs and toss to coat.
3. Add the ground turkey and mix well.
4. Transfer into a 1½-quart casserole or large loaf pan. Bake, uncovered,
   in a 350-degree oven for 55-60 minutes or until no longer pink and
   internal temperature on a meat thermometer is 170 degrees.
5. Serve with ketchup or steak sauce, if desired.

Makes 6 servings.

Serving suggestion: Serve with mashed potatoes, Green Bean Amandine (page
189), and warm gluten-free bread.

Ground Turkey Meatloaf Patties: Prepare as above through step 3, and then
form into 6 patties. Fry in a lightly oiled pan for 5-10 minutes, turning once or until
no longer pink and internal temperature on a meat thermometer is 170 degrees.

Stuffing (Corn Bread) EZ

Ingredients

8 slices uncooked bacon, chopped (4 ounces)
1½ cup chopped celery (3 large stalks)
1½ cup chopped onion (1 large)
2 eggs, beaten
1 tablespoon dried parsley, crushed
1 teaspoon poultry seasoning
6 cups corn bread, cooled and coarsely crumbled (page 51)
½ to ¾ cup chicken broth (4-6 ounces)

Directions

1. In a frying pan, combine the bacon, celery, and onion. Fry on medium heat until the bacon is crisp and the onions are translucent.
2. Meanwhile, in a bowl, combine the eggs, parsley, and poultry seasoning.
3. Place the cornbread crumbs in a large mixing bowl. Add the egg mixture and toss. Add the bacon mixture, including the bacon drippings. Toss. Add enough of the chicken broth to lightly moisten; do not use too much.

Makes enough stuffing for a 10-pound turkey or domestic goose.

To bake separately: Pour the stuffing into 13 x 9 x 2-inch baking pan, being careful not to mash the stuffing in too tight. Bake in a 350-degree oven for 30-40 minutes or until internal temperature reaches 165 degrees.

Note: To make this recipe with bread cubes, substitute 3 cups dried gluten-free bread cubes plus one half of the recipe for cornbread, crumbled. Allow the bread cubes to completely dry out or use less broth. (To make the bread cubes, toast the bread and slice into ½ - to 1-inch cubes.)

Stuffing (Traditional) EZ

Ingredients

1 cup chopped onion (1 medium)
1 cup chopped celery (2 large stalks)
¼ cup margarine or butter (½ stick)
2 eggs, beaten
½ teaspoon poultry seasoning
1 tablespoon dried parsley, crushed
4 cups dried gluten-free bread cubes
⅓ to ½ cup chicken broth

Directions

1. In a frying pan, combine the onion, celery, and margarine. Cook until tender and the onion is translucent.
2. Meanwhile, in a large bowl, combine the eggs, poultry seasoning, and parsley. Add the onion mixture and stir to combine.
3. Add the dried bread cubes and toss to combine. Add the broth, 1 tablespoon at a time, just enough to moisten, tossing gently.

Makes enough dressing to stuff a 4-5 pound chicken. Double the recipe to stuff an 8-10 pound turkey.

To bake separately: Pour the dressing into a 13 x 9 x 2-inch baking pan, being careful not to mash it in too tight. Bake in a 350-degree oven for 20-30 minutes or until internal temperature reaches 165 degrees.

"Any idiot can handle a crisis;
it's this day-to-day living that wears you out."
—Anton Chekhov

Pizza

Mini Pizzas

My daughter requested this recipe. We think she had a great idea!

Ingredients

1 Buttermilk Biscuit Recipe (page 50)
¼ cup Pizza Sauce (next page)
24 slices of pepperoni
3 cups shredded Mozzarella
½ cup sliced black olives, drained (4-ounce can)*(optional)*

Directions   ***Preheat oven to 450 degrees.***

1. Place one heaping tablespoon of the biscuit dough in the bottom of each of 24 well-greased muffin cups.
2. Top the dough with one slice of pepperoni, pressing down slightly to form the crust around the pepperoni.
3. Drop ½ teaspoon pizza sauce and 2 tablespoons shredded cheese on each biscuit. Place one olive slice on top of each biscuit.
4. Bake in 450-degree oven for 11-13 minutes.

Makes 8 servings of 3 mini pizzas.

Pizza Sauce

If you choose to make your own pizza sauce, here's one that's great to keep in a squeeze bottle so your child can have a quick pizza nearly anytime!

Ingredients

1 15-ounce can tomato sauce
1 teaspoon sugar* *(optional)*
½ teaspoon garlic powder
2 teaspoons dried basil, crushed
1 teaspoon dried oregano, crushed
1 teaspoon dried minced onion

Directions

1. Place all the ingredients in a medium saucepan. Bring to a boil. Reduce heat, cover, and simmer for 10 minutes.
2. Spoon the sauce onto a prepared pizza crust, or cool and store in a squeeze bottle in the refrigerator for up to 2 weeks.

Makes enough sauce for 2 full-sized pizzas.

---

* The sugar reduces the acidity of the tomato sauce.

Quick Lunch Pizza

Ingredients

1 corn or Mock Flour Tortilla (page 53)
2 tablespoons pizza sauce (see previous recipe)
Toppings of your choice
½ cup mozzarella cheese

Directions

1. Place the tortilla on a microwave-safe plate.
2. Spread the pizza sauce on the tortilla, to within ½ inch of the edge.
3. Top with your favorite toppings (or leftover meats, etc.). Sprinkle with the cheese.
4. Microwave on high for 1 minute or until the cheese is melted and the toppings are hot. Cut into quarters.

Makes one serving.

Traditional Pizza Crust

My family has used this recipe more than any other recipe in the book. We usually make this recipe every Saturday! For best results, use a heavy-duty mixer with a flat beater attachment.

Ingredients

1½ cups rice flour
1 cup tapioca flour
½ cup potato starch flour
1 tablespoon xanthan gum
¼ teaspoon salt
1 teaspoon unflavored gelatin
1 package (2¼ teaspoons) dry yeast
1 cup water
2 tablespoons cooking oil
1 teaspoon vinegar
1 large egg, room temperature

Directions   *Preheat oven to 425 degrees.*

1. Combine rice flour, tapioca flour, potato starch flour, xanthan gum, salt, unflavored gelatin, and dry yeast in a large bowl.
2. In a saucepan (or microwave) heat the water to 120 to 130 degrees on a candy thermometer. Remove from heat.
3. Add the cooking oil to the water.
4. With an electric mixer on low (or a heavy-duty mixer on slow), slowly add the water/oil mixture to the dry ingredients. Then add the vinegar, followed by the egg. Beat the dough on high-speed of electric mixer for three minutes (on medium for the heavy-duty mixer.)

Family-size Pizza: Cover two ungreased cookie sheets with a sheet of parchment paper, trimming the edges as needed. Spread out half of the dough on each. Cover with slightly oiled parchment paper, wax paper, or plastic wrap. With hands (or small pizza rolling pin), press out into 10- to 12-inch circles, making the edges slightly thicker to hold the sauce and toppings in. Remove the oiled cover.

   a. Bake crusts on the lined cookie sheet for eight minutes in preheated 425-degree oven.

   b. Remove crusts from oven. Top the hot crusts with about ½-cup pizza sauce each. Add the toppings of your choice, such as pepperoni and mozzarella cheese.

   c. Bake an additional 15-20 minutes or until crust is crisp and lightly browned, and cheese is melted.

Makes 8 two-piece servings.

Individual-size Pizza: Prepare as above, except spread out the pizza dough into 4- to 5-inch circles on a greased or parchment-lined cookie sheet. Or, for added fun, shape the individual crusts into your child's favorite shapes: squares, triangles, cars, boats, snowman, tree, cat's head, Mickey Mouse, etc.

   a. Bake crusts for eight minutes in preheated 425-degree oven.

   b. Remove crusts from oven. Top the hot crusts with about 3 tablespoons pizza sauce each. Add the toppings of your choice, such as pepperoni and mozzarella cheese.

   c. Bake an additional 10-15 minutes or until crust is crisp and lightly browned, and cheese is melted.

Makes 8 individual serving pizzas.

Stuffed Crust Pizza: Place a piece of parchment paper on the pizza pan or cookie sheet (but do not trim). Press or roll out pizza dough to 12 to14-inch circles on pans.

   a. Tear a piece of mozzarella string cheese lengthwise into three strips. Arrange the strips of cheese one-inch from the edge of the crust. Repeat with additional strips of string cheese until the crust is encircled.

   b. Using the lower parchment paper as a guide, roll the outer inch of dough over the string cheese strips. Press the seam closed with fingers.

   c. Trim extra parchment paper with scissors then bake crust for 8 minutes. Remove from oven, add toppings of your choice, and bake an additional 15-20 minutes.

Makes 8 two-piece servings.

Yeast-Free Bean Flour Pizza Crust

A light, crispy crust that your whole family, if not the entire neighborhood, will enjoy!

Ingredients

¼ cup light bean flour
½ cup tapioca flour
½ cup brown rice flour
¼ cup rice flour
1 teaspoon baking powder
¼ teaspoon salt
¼ cup vegetable oil
½ cup milk or non-dairy creamer
Pizza sauce
Toppings of choice

Directions
Preheat oven to 400 degrees.

1. Combine bean, tapioca, brown rice, and rice flours, baking powder, and salt in a medium-sized bowl.
2. In a smaller bowl or liquid measuring cup, mix the oil and the milk together. Add to the dry ingredients and mix well.
3. On a greased cookie sheet, spread out the dough. Cover with oiled waxed paper or plastic wrap. With hands, press out into a 10- to 12-inch circle, making the edges slightly thicker to hold the sauce and toppings in.
4. Bake for 10 minutes at 400 degrees. Remove crust from the oven.
5. Top the hot crust with about ½ cup pizza sauce. Add the toppings of your choice, such as pepperoni and mozzarella cheese. Bake an additional 9-10 minutes.

Makes 4 two-piece servings.

Individual Pizzas: Prepare as above through step 2. On a greased cookie sheet spread out ¼ cup of the dough and cover with oiled wax paper or plastic wrap. With hands, spread out into a 4- to 5-inch circle, making the edges slightly thicker to hold the toppings in. Repeat with the rest of the dough. Continue with step 4. Makes 4 individual pizzas.

To Freeze for Later Use: Prepare the pizza crusts as above, except press the crusts out between two pieces of oiled wax paper or plastic wrap. Stack the crusts, separated by the waxed paper or plastic wrap, on top of one another. Put into a large zip-style freezer bag, label, and freeze. To use, defrost on the counter for 20-30 minutes or defrost in the microwave.

Yeast-Free Individual Pizza Crust

This recipe is included for children who do not tolerate yeast. These crusts do well in a toaster oven for a quick lunch, or whenever you need them.

Ingredients

1 cup rice flour
¾ cup potato starch flour
¾ cup tapioca flour
½ cup dry milk powder or substitute
1 tablespoon baking powder
½ teaspoon salt
2 tablespoons shortening
¾ cup water

Directions

1. In a mixing bowl, combine the rice flour, potato starch flour, tapioca flour, milk powder, baking powder, and salt. Add the shortening. With a pastry blender or your fingers, mix until crumbly.
2. Pour in the water and mix until the dough clings together.
3. Divide the dough into 8 pieces. (Cover the pieces you are not working on with a damp cloth or plastic wrap to prevent over-drying.)
4. Place a piece of dough on a lightly oiled cookie sheet and cover lightly with a lightly oiled piece of waxed paper or plastic wrap. Press out the dough with your hands, from the center outward, into a circle 4 to 5 inches in diameter and about ¼ inch thick. Remove the waxed paper and push up the edges slightly to contain the sauce and fillings. Repeat the above procedure with the other 7 pieces to bake immediately, or see note below for baking later.
5. Bake prepared crusts in a preheated 400 degree oven for 5 minutes.
6. Remove crusts from the oven. Spread with 2-3 tablespoons of pizza sauce (recipe page 147), or other desired sauce and toppings. Sprinkle with ¼ to ½ cup of mozzarella cheese.

7. Return pizza to oven for 7 to 10 minutes, or until cheese is melted and the crust is golden brown.

Makes 8 individual pizzas.

To Freeze for Later Use: Press the dough out between two pieces of lightly oiled waxed paper and stack until all crusts are completed. To freeze the crusts, leave oiled waxed paper between them and place in zipper-style freezer bags. Label and date, then freeze. To prepare, remove the required crusts from the freezer and defrost on the counter for 20-30 minutes or in the microwave on defrost for 45 to 60 seconds. After defrosting, place on lightly oiled cookie sheet, push the edges up slightly, and continue as above with step 5.

"Things do not change; we change."
—Henry David Thoreau

Pasta & Rice

Baked Macaroni-N-Cheese

Ingredients

1 16-ounce package rice/corn macaroni (4½ cups)
2 tablespoons margarine or butter
3 tablespoons rice flour
2½ cups milk
2 cups cubed American cheese
2 cups shredded cheddar cheese
½ cup grated Parmesan cheese (2 ounces)

Topping

½ cup shredded cheddar cheese
¼ cup grated Parmesan cheese (1 ounce)

Directions   *Preheat oven to 350 degrees.*

1. Cook macaroni according to package directions. Drain and rinse well.
2. Meanwhile, melt the margarine in a medium-sized saucepan. Add rice flour and stir for 15 seconds.
3. Add milk all at once. Heat on high until boiling. Reduce heat and stir often until slightly thickened.
4. Add the 2 cups American cheese, the 2 cups cheddar cheese, and ½ cup Parmesan cheese to the milk mixture, stirring until melted.
5. Add cooked macaroni to cheese mixture and stir.
6. Transfer to a 2-quart casserole dish. Top with the ½ cup cheddar and ¼ cup Parmesan cheeses.
7. Bake in 350-degree oven for 30 minutes or until bubbly and top is slightly browned. Let stand for 10 minutes before serving.

Makes 8 servings.

Fresh Egg Pasta

Ingredients

1 cup tapioca flour
1 cup rice flour
⅔ cup potato starch flour
⅓ cup light bean flour
½ teaspoon salt
1 teaspoon xanthan gum
1 teaspoon oil
4 eggs, beaten
⅓ cup water

Directions

1. Combine the tapioca flour, rice flour, potato starch flour, light bean flour, salt, and xanthan gum.
2. Make a well in the center of the dry ingredients by pushing to the sides of the bowl with a spoon or spatula. Add the oil and the eggs. Combine the flour mixture and egg mixture with a fork or pastry blender. Add one tablespoon of water at a time, combining the dough with the fork or pastry blender after each addition.
3. Combine and knead the dough on a rice-floured surface for about five minutes or until smooth.
4. Cover the dough and set it aside for 10 minutes.
5. Divide the dough into four pieces. (Refrigerate remaining ¾ of the dough until ready to use.) Use one of the cutting methods listed below.
   - On a lightly rice-floured surface roll the first piece of dough to about ¹⁄₁₆ th of an inch thick and about 12 x 12-inches square. Let stand for 20 minutes. Cut dough into desired shapes.
   - If using a pasta machine, pass the dough through the machine according to the manufacturer's directions until ¹⁄₁₆ of an inch thick. Let stand for 20 minutes. Then cut as desired. (**Note**: This will *have* to be a gluten-free dedicated machine as the glutens will be impossible to remove from the machine in between batches.)

6. To cook the pasta, measure 3 quarts of water for every 4-8 ounces of pasta into a large saucepan or Dutch oven. Bring water to a boil and, if desired, add a teaspoon salt and a tablespoon olive oil or cooking oil to help keep the pasta from sticking.
7. Add the pasta a little at a time so the water does not stop boiling. (Long pastas, such as spaghetti, will need to be held at one end and dipped gently into the water. As the pasta softens, gently curl the pasta around the pan and down into the water.)
8. Reduce the heat slightly and boil uncovered, for the time specified below or until the pasta is tender but still firm. Stir occasionally. Test often for doneness near the end of the cooking time.
9. Drain in a colander.

Makes 1 pound of fresh pasta (8 servings).

PASTA SHAPE ...... COOKING TIME*

Noodles/Fettuccine/Linguine/Spaghetti ...... 1½ to 2 minutes
Bow Ties/Manicotti/Lasagna ...... 2 to 3 minutes
Ravioli ...... 6 to 8 minutes
Tortellini ...... 8 to 10 minutes

* *If the pasta is being cooked frozen, allow a few more minutes. Drying completely is not recommended.*

Storage: Let dry on a wire rack for about one hour before storing. Place in an airtight container for up to 3 days in the refrigerator or 6 months in the freezer.

Noodles in Alfredo Sauce

Ingredients

8 ounces (about 2¼ cups) gluten-free noodles
2 tablespoons margarine or butter
1-2 cloves garlic, minced (as desired)
⅔ cup Parmesan cheese (2⅔ ounces)
1½ cups (12 ounces) light cream or whipping cream, room temperature

Directions

1. Cook noodles according to package directions. Drain and rinse in hot water.
2. Add margarine and garlic to noodle pan and heat for about a minute until the margarine is melted and the garlic softens. Add Parmesan cheese and cream. Stir until combined and heat until slightly thickened.
3. Remove sauce from heat. Add noodles and toss well.

Makes 4 servings.

Chicken and Alfredo Sauce: Add 1 cup cooked, cubed chicken and ½ cup thinly sliced, lightly sautéed zucchini, if desired.

Brown Rice Pilaf

Ingredients

   2 tablespoons cooking oil
   3 cups brown rice, uncooked
   ¼ cup sesame seeds (about 1 ounce)
   1 cup finely chopped celery (2 stalks)
   ½ cup chopped red bell pepper (½ medium) *(optional)*
   1 cup chopped green bell pepper (1 medium)
   ¼ cup finely chopped onion (½ medium) *(optional)*
   1 tablespoon parsley
   1 teaspoon garlic powder
   1 teaspoon turmeric

Directions

1. In a large saucepan, combine cooking oil, brown rice, sesame seeds, celery, red bell pepper, if used, green bell pepper, and onion, if used. Heat and stir until brown rice has browned and onion is translucent, about 2 minutes.
2. Add parsley, garlic powder, turmeric, and 6 cups of water. Heat to boiling. Cover and simmer for 40 minutes or until all liquid is absorbed.

Makes 12 (½ cup) servings.

Curried Rice Mix

Ingredients

1 cup white rice, uncooked
2 teaspoons chicken or vegetable bouillon granules (2 cubes)
½ -1 teaspoon curry powder (to taste)
1 tablespoon minced dried onion
½ teaspoon ground cumin
½ teaspoon parsley flakes
½ teaspoon salt or celery salt
2 tablespoons margarine or butter

Directions

1. In a large saucepan, combine rice, bouillon cubes, curry powder, onion, cumin, parsley flakes, salt or celery salt, margarine, and 2 cups of water. Heat to boiling.
2. Cover and simmer for 20 minutes or until all liquid is absorbed.
3. Fluff with a fork before serving.

Makes 4 (½ cup) side dish servings.

Herb Rice

Ingredients

1 cup white rice, uncooked
2 teaspoons beef or vegetable bouillon granules (2 cubes)
1 tablespoon ground onion flakes *(optional)*
½ teaspoon rosemary
½ teaspoon marjoram or oregano
½ teaspoon thyme leaves
½ teaspoon salt or celery salt
2 tablespoons margarine or butter

Directions

1. In a large saucepan, combine rice, bouillon cubes, onion flakes, rosemary, marjoram or oregano, thyme, salt or celery salt, margarine, and 2 cups of water. Heat to boiling.
2. Cover and simmer for 20 minutes or until all liquid is absorbed.
3. Fluff with a fork before serving.

Makes 4 (½ cup) side dish servings.

Rice for Beef or Pork

Ingredients

    1½ cups long grain rice, uncooked
    3 teaspoons beef bouillon granules (3 cubes)
    1 teaspoon dried basil
    1 bay leaf

Directions

1. Place rice, bouillon, basil, bay leaf, and 3 cups of water in a large saucepan. Cover and bring to a boil.
2. Reduce heat and simmer for 20 minutes or until water is absorbed and the rice is tender. (Do not remove lid until water appears absorbed.)
3. Remove bay leaf.
4. Fluff with a fork before serving.

Makes 6 servings.

Rice for Chicken

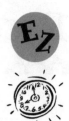

Ingredients

1½ cups long grain rice, uncooked
3 teaspoons chicken bouillon granules (3 cubes)
¼ teaspoon poultry seasoning

Directions

1. Place rice, bouillon, poultry seasoning, and 3 cups water in a large saucepan. Cover and bring to a boil.
2. Reduce heat and simmer for 20 minutes or until water is absorbed and the rice is tender. (Do not remove lid until water appears absorbed.)
3. Fluff with a fork before serving.

Makes 6 servings.

Rosemary Rice Mix

Ingredients

1 cup white rice, uncooked
1 teaspoon chicken bouillon granules (1 cube)
¾ teaspoon poultry seasoning
¼ teaspoon rosemary, crushed
¼ teaspoon basil, crushed
¼ teaspoon celery seed
2 tablespoons margarine or butter

Directions

1. In a large saucepan, combine rice, bouillon cubes, poultry seasoning, rosemary, basil, celery seed, margarine, and 2 cups of water. Heat to boiling.
2. Cover and simmer for 20 minutes or until all liquid is absorbed.
3. Fluff with a fork before serving.

Makes 4 (½ cup) side dish servings.

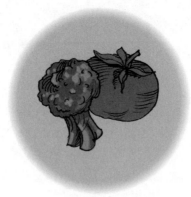

Salads & Vegetables

Salads & Dressings ❦ Vegetables

"Life itself is a race, marked by a start, and a finish.

It is what we learn during the race, and how we apply it,

that determines whether our participation

has had particular value.

If we learn from each success, and each failure,

and improve ourselves through this process,

then, at the end, we will have fulfilled

our potential and performed well."

—Dr. Ferdinand Porsche

*"We are here to add what we can to life,
not to get what we can from it."*
—William Osler

Salads & Dressings

Apple Salad

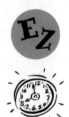

Ingredients

½ cup mayonnaise or plain yogurt
1 teaspoon lemon juice
2 medium apples, chopped (2 cups)
½ cup raisins
½ large stalk of celery, chopped (½ cup)
½ cup walnuts or pecans, chopped *(optional)*
½ cup mini marshmallows *(optional)*

Directions

1. In a medium-sized bowl, combine the mayonnaise and lemon juice.
2. Add the apple, raisins, celery, and walnuts, if desired. Mix well.
3. Add the mini marshmallows, if desired.

Makes 6 ½-cup servings.

Creamy Coleslaw

Ingredients

1 head cabbage, 1½ pounds (7 cups shredded)
2 medium carrots (¾ cup shredded)
1 cup gluten-free mayonnaise or substitute
2 tablespoons apple cider vinegar
1 tablespoon sugar
1 teaspoon celery seeds
¼ teaspoon sesame oil *(optional)*
½ cup raisins or Craisins® dried cranberries *(optional)*
2 tablespoons sesame seeds

Directions

1. In a large mixing bowl, combine the cabbage and carrots. Set aside.
2. In a medium-sized bowl, combine the mayonnaise, apple cider vinegar, sugar, celery seed, and sesame oil, if used. Add raisins, if used, and sesame seeds.
3. Pour the mayonnaise mixture over the cabbage mixture and toss well to coat. Chill 1-24 hours before serving.
4. Garnish with a parsley twig and ground paprika, if desired.

Makes 16 side dish servings.

Variations:

- Substitute a 16-ounce package of coleslaw salad mix for the cabbage and shredded carrots.
- Omit sesame oil and substitute ½ cup chopped walnuts, pecans, almonds, or roasted pine nuts for the sesame seeds.
- For a sugar-free salad, substitute 3 packages of Splenda® sweetener for the sugar.

Creamy Pasta Salad

Ingredients

2¼ cups gluten-free macaroni or Rotini, uncooked (8 ounces)
3 tablespoons carrot, peeled and shredded (1 medium)
¼ cup celery, chopped (1 stalk)
½ cup mayonnaise or substitute
1 teaspoon gluten-free prepared mustard
½ teaspoon celery seed

Directions

1. Cook macaroni according to package directions. Drain in a colander and rinse with hot water for 30 seconds. Rinse with cold water for 2 minutes or until cool.
2. Meanwhile, in a medium-sized bowl, combine the carrot, celery, mayonnaise, mustard, and celery seed.
3. Add cooled pasta to vegetable mixture and toss. Sprinkle with salt and pepper, if desired. Cover and refrigerate 1 to 14 hours before serving. Sprinkle with bacon bits, if desired.

Makes 4-5 servings.

Creamy Potato Salad

Ingredients

5-6 large potatoes (7-8 medium)
2 stalks celery, chopped (½ cup)
⅓ cup chopped onion (if desired)
1 cup gluten-free mayonnaise or substitute
1 tablespoon apple cider or other vinegar
2 teaspoons gluten-free prepared mustard
¼ teaspoon ground pepper
½ teaspoon celery seeds

Directions

1. Wash and cook unpeeled potatoes in boiling water for 20 minutes. Drain and cool. When cool, peel (if desired) and cut into cubes. Set aside.
2. In a large bowl, combine celery, onion, mayonnaise, apple cider vinegar, mustard, ground pepper, and celery seeds.
3. Add the cooled potatoes and toss to coat.
4. Cover with plastic wrap or tight-fitting lid. Chill for 2 to 24 hours before serving.

Makes 16 ½-cup servings.

Variations: Add ½ small green pepper, finely chopped.
Add ½ small sweet red pepper, finely chopped.
Add 2 tablespoons sweet or dill relish.
Add ½ cup sliced black olives, drained.
Replace the onion with green onions.
Replace the mustard with Dijon mustard.

Macaroni Salad

Ingredients

2¼ cups gluten-free macaroni or Rotini (8 ounces)
½ cup celery, chopped (2 stalks)
⅓ cup onion, chopped (½ small)
2 tablespoons sweet or dill relish
¼ cup sliced black olives (4 ounces, drained)
⅓ cup mayonnaise or substitute
⅓ cup sour cream or substitute
1 teaspoon prepared mustard
½ teaspoon celery seeds
1 cup cherry tomatoes, halved *(optional)*

Directions

1. Cook pasta according to package directions. Drain and rinse with cool water. Let cool completely.
2. In a large bowl, combine the celery, onion, relish, black olives, mayonnaise, sour cream, mustard, and celery seeds. Mix well.
3. Add the cooled pasta and toss well to coat.
4. Cover and refrigerate at least 1 hour.
5. Garnish with the cherry tomatoes, if desired.

Makes 8 servings.

Sesame Chicken Salad

Ingredients

1 skinless, boneless chicken breast
1 tablespoon cooking oil
3 tablespoons orange juice
1 tablespoon honey
1 teaspoon gluten-free soy sauce
¼ teaspoon grated ginger root
¼ teaspoon sesame oil
1 recipe Creamy Coleslaw (page 171)

Directions

1. Cut the chicken breast into bite-sized pieces.
2. In a small frying pan, cook the chicken pieces with ½ cup water, adding water as needed until chicken is done.
3. Add the cooking oil. Brown the chicken pieces.
4. Meanwhile, in a small bowl, combine orange juice, honey, soy sauce, ginger root, and sesame oil.
5. Add to the chicken pieces. Cook on low until bubbly (about 30 seconds). Remove from heat, set aside to cool.
6. Prepare the Creamy Coleslaw.
7. Add the chicken pieces to the Creamy Coleslaw. Serve immediately or chill for 1 to 24 hours.

Makes 4 main-dish servings.

Tuna Salad

Ingredients

½ cup mayonnaise or substitute
1 tablespoon sweet or dilled pickle relish
2¼ cups tuna, drained (12-14 ounces)
¼ cup walnuts, chopped *(optional)*

Directions

In a medium-sized bowl, combine the mayonnaise, pickle relish, tuna, and walnuts.

Makes 4 servings.

Ham Salad: Prepare as above, substituting diced or minced ham for the tuna.

Chicken Salad: Prepare as above, substituting diced or minced chicken (perhaps leftover from a previous meal) or drained canned chicken.

Egg Salad: Prepare as above, omitting walnuts and substituting 6 hard cooked eggs, peeled, cooled, and diced.

Serving suggestions: Serve on a bed of lettuce with tomato slices or serve on gluten-free bread (see Breads, pages 45-85) as a sandwich or on crackers with cheese slices.

Buttermilk Dressing

Ingredients

½ cup cottage cheese

1 cup mayonnaise (8 ounces)

2 tablespoons powdered cultured buttermilk

½ cup milk

¼ cup grated Parmesan cheese

1 teaspoon dried dill weed, crushed

1 teaspoon dried parsley, crushed

¼ teaspoon garlic powder

¼ teaspoon dried, granulated onion

Directions

1. In a blender or food processor, whip the cottage cheese until smooth.
2. Add the mayonnaise, buttermilk powder, and milk. Blend for 30 seconds.
3. Add the Parmesan cheese, dill weed, parsley, garlic powder, and granulated onion. Blend for 1 minute.
4. Chill for at least 2 hours before serving. Store in the refrigerator for up to two weeks.

Makes 36 2-tablespoon servings.

Cream Cheese Fruit Dressing

A tasty dip for fresh fruit or topping for canned fruit.

Ingredients

1 3-ounce package cream cheese
2-4 tablespoons juice (orange, lemon, apricot nectar, pineapple, etc.)

Directions

1. In a small bowl, beat the cream cheese with an electric mixer until smooth.
2. Add the juice 1 tablespoon at a time, beating between additions, until desired consistency and flavor.

Makes 6 1-tablespoon servings.

Store in the refrigerator for up to 10 days.

Variation: Replace the juice with milk and add ½ teaspoon ground cinnamon and 1 tablespoon sugar.

Dilly Vegetable Dip

Ingredients

　　1 3-ounce package cream cheese
　　1 teaspoon lemon juice
　　2-4 tablespoons milk
　　1-2 tablespoons dried dill weed

Directions

1. In a small bowl, beat the cream cheese with an electric mixer until smooth.
2. Add the lemon juice and milk 1 tablespoon at a time, beating between additions, until desired consistency. Add the dill until desired flavor.

Makes 6 1-tablespoon servings.

Store in the refrigerator for up to 10 days.

Serving suggestion: Use as a dip for carrot sticks, celery, tomato slices, etc.

Lemon Yogurt Fruit Dressing

Ingredients

¾ cup lemon yogurt (6 ounces)
½ cup frozen whipped cream topping, thawed (or Mock Whip Cream, page 239)
½ teaspoon lemon zest
1-3 tablespoons lemon juice

Directions

1. In a cooled bowl, combine the lemon yogurt, whipped topping, and lemon zest with an electric mixer.
2. Add lemon juice, one teaspoon at a time, beating after each addition, until the desired consistency.

Makes 1¼ cups (20 1-tablespoon servings).

Serving suggestion: Use as a dip for strawberries, apples, and banana slices.

"A food is not necessarily essential just because your child hates it."
—Katherine Whitehorn

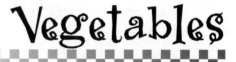

Baked French Fries

Ingredients

4 medium potatoes
4 tablespoons margarine or butter

Directions

Preheat oven to 450 degrees.

1. Peel or wash the potatoes. Cut the potatoes lengthwise into strips ½- to ¾-inch wide. Rinse and drain well.
2. Place the margarine in a shallow baking pan (15 x 10 x 1). Put in the oven to melt. Remove from the oven.
3. Arrange the potatoes in a single layer in the baking pan. Bake in a 450-degree oven for 25-30 minutes or until browned. Sprinkle with salt or seasoned salt, if desired.

Makes 4 servings.

Baked Garlic Parmesan Fries

Ingredients

6 medium potatoes
6 tablespoons margarine or butter
½ teaspoon garlic powder
2 tablespoons dried parsley, crushed
¼ cup potato starch flour
½ cup grated Parmesan cheese (2 ounces)

Directions

Preheat oven to 450 degrees.

1. Peel or wash the potatoes. Cut the potatoes lengthwise into ½- to ¾-inch wide strips. Rinse and drain well.
2. Place the margarine in a shallow baking pan (15 x 10 x 1). Put in the oven to melt. Remove from the oven.
3. In a large plastic zip-style bag, combine the garlic powder, parsley, potato starch flour, and the grated Parmesan, shaking to mix well.
4. Add about one-sixth of the potato strips to the bag and shake to coat. Remove the coated potatoes, gently shaking off excess coating and place in the shallow baking pan in a single layer. Continue with the remaining potatoes.
5. Bake at 450 degrees for 25-35 minutes or until golden brown and tender. (Do not turn the fries during baking.)

Makes 6 servings.

Baked Potatoes

Ingredients

4 medium-sized baking potatoes
2 tablespoons margarine or butter

Directions   *Preheat oven to 425 degrees.*

1. Wash potatoes and scrub well. Prick several times with a fork.
2. Rub each potato with ½ tablespoon of the margarine or butter.
3. Bake in a 425-degree oven for 40-50 minutes or until tender.
4. Remove from oven. Wrap with a hot pad or towel and pat firmly to loosen potato from skin. Make a cut through the length of the potato and press both ends slightly together to open the cut. Top with margarine, butter, sour cream, shredded cheese, or any other favorite topping.

Makes 4 servings.

Variation: Substitute sweet potatoes or yams for the baking potatoes.

Barbeque Butter Beans

Ingredients

2 cups butter beans (or lima), fresh or frozen
6 slices bacon or turkey bacon (¼ pound)
¼ cup finely chopped onion (or 1 tablespoon dried minced onion)
½ cup finely chopped bell pepper (*optional*)
2 tablespoons vinegar
1 cup ketchup (8 ounces)
½ cup molasses or maple syrup (4 ounces)
2 tablespoons Worcestershire sauce
1 teaspoon dry mustard
¼ teaspoon celery seed
1 tablespoon packed brown sugar (*optional*)
½ teaspoon salt
½ teaspoon pepper

Directions

1. Bring 6 cups of water to a boil in a large saucepan. Add the butter beans. Return to a boil. Cover and reduce heat. Simmer for 40-50 minutes or until tender.
2. Meanwhile, in a large frying pan, cook the bacon until crisp. Remove the bacon from the pan and drain on paper towels. Reserve 1 tablespoon of the drippings (or all of the drippings, if using turkey bacon). Crumble the bacon and set aside.
3. In the same pan, cook the onion and bell pepper in reserved drippings, until tender and onion is translucent, not brown.
4. In a mixing bowl, combine the vinegar, ketchup, molasses, Worcestershire sauce, dry mustard, celery seed, brown sugar (if used), salt, and pepper. Set aside.
5. Reserving ½ cup of the liquid, drain the cooked butter beans. Return the butter beans and the reserved liquid to the pan. Add the molasses mixture and stir. Cook the beans on low for an additional 15 minutes or until desired consistency.
6. Remove from heat. Top with reserved crumbled bacon.

Makes 6 servings.

Broccoli with Cheese Sauce

Ingredients

6 cups broccoli, cut up (1½ pounds) or 16-ounce package frozen
1 tablespoon margarine or butter
2 tablespoons sweet rice flour or white rice flour
1¼ cups milk
1½ cups shredded cheddar cheese (6 ounces)
½ cup shredded Monterey Jack cheese or mozzarella cheese (2 ounces)
¼ cup grated Parmesan cheese

Directions

1. Cook fresh broccoli, covered, in a small amount of boiling water for 9-11 minutes or until tender. (Or follow package directions, if frozen.)
2. Meanwhile, melt margarine in a medium-sized saucepan. Add the sweet rice flour and stir for 15 seconds. Add the milk all at once. Heat on high until boiling. Reduce heat and stir continuously until slightly thickened.
3. Add cheddar cheese, Monterey Jack cheese, and Parmesan cheese. Stir until cheeses are melted and smooth. Remove from heat and cover.
4. Drain the cooked broccoli. Spoon the cheese sauce over the broccoli or pass the cheese sauce when serving the broccoli.

Makes 6 servings.

Variations: Substitute cauliflower, green beans, asparagus, turnips, or parsnips for the broccoli.

Creamy Green Bean Casserole

Ingredients

1 tablespoon margarine or butter

2 tablespoons sweet rice flour or white rice flour

1¼ cups milk or milk substitute

½ cup sour cream or milk-free substitute

2 cups French-style green beans (16-ounce can, drained, or 9-ounce package frozen)

¼ cup crushed sour cream and onion potato chips

Directions

Preheat oven to 350 degrees.

1. Melt margarine in a medium-sized saucepan. Add the sweet rice flour and stir for 15 seconds. Add milk all at once. Heat on high until boiling. Reduce heat and stir continually until slightly thickened. Remove from heat.

2. Add sour cream and stir. Add green beans and stir to combine.

3. Transfer mixture to a 1-quart casserole dish. Bake in a 350-degree oven for 20-25 minutes or until bubbly. Remove from oven.

4. Sprinkle the top of the casserole with the sour cream and onion potato chip crumbs. Return to oven and bake for 5 additional minutes or until chips are lightly browned.

Makes 4 servings.

Easy Baked Beans

Ingredients

3 slices of bacon, uncooked
½ cup chopped onion (½ medium)
3½ cups canned pinto beans (29 ounces)
½ cup ketchup (4 ounces)
⅓ cup packed brown sugar or molasses
2 tablespoons maple syrup
2 teaspoons yellow mustard
1½ teaspoons Worcestershire sauce
1 teaspoon apple cider vinegar

Directions
Preheat oven to 350 degrees.

1. In a skillet, fry the bacon until crisp. Remove the bacon and reserve 1½ teaspoons of the drippings. Drain and crumble the bacon. Set aside.
2. Cook the onion in the reserved drippings until the onion is translucent, not brown.
3. In a 2-quart casserole dish, combine the cooked onion, beans, ketchup, brown sugar or molasses, maple syrup, mustard, Worcestershire sauce, and apple cider vinegar.
4. Bake in a 350-degree oven for 1 hour. Remove from oven and sprinkle bacon pieces on top of beans. Return to oven and bake an additional 10 minutes.

Stovetop Directions

Follow recipe through step 2 and then substitute a 2-quart saucepan for the casserole dish. Simmer on the stovetop over medium heat for 15 minutes. Add the bacon and simmer for 5 minutes more. (The flavor is not quite as good as the baked version, but it works great if you are pinched for time!)

Green Bean Amandine

Ingredients

2 cups French-style green beans (16-ounce can, drained,
or 9-ounce package frozen)
1 tablespoon margarine or butter
½ cup slivered or sliced almonds (3 ounces)
1-2 teaspoons lemon juice

Directions

1. Cook green beans according to package directions.
2. Meanwhile, melt margarine in a small omelet pan or saucepan. Add
   the almonds, stirring frequently until lightly browned. Add lemon
   juice according to taste, stir, and remove from heat.
3. Drain cooked green beans (if necessary). Add to almond mixture. Toss
   to combine.

Makes 4 servings.

Spaghetti Squash

Adds a vegetable to dinner without the fuss.

Ingredients

1 spaghetti squash (1½-2 pounds)

Directions   *Preheat oven to 350 degrees.*

1. Cut the squash lengthwise. Remove the seeds and discard. Rinse squash in cold water and sprinkle with salt, if desired.
2. Place squash halves, cut side down in a shallow baking dish. Add ½ inch of water to the dish.
3. Bake in a 350-degree oven for 1 hour or until soft.
4. Remove from oven. Run a fork lengthwise through the cooked squash to release the strands of squash from the skin. Season as desired or choose from the suggestions below.

Makes 4 servings.

Serving suggestions:

- Top with butter or oil and freshly chopped herbs, such as minced garlic, fresh basil, fresh dill, chopped chives, etc.
- Serve with spaghetti sauce, as with traditional pasta.
- Serve with Parmesan cheese, minced garlic, and butter or oil.

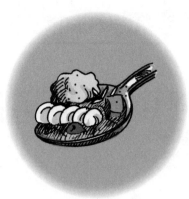

Soups & Stews

"Cooking is like love.

It should be entered into

with abandon or not at all."

—Harriet Van Horne

Chicken and Dumplings

Ingredients

2½-3 pounds broiler-fryer chicken, cut up
½ teaspoon poultry seasoning
¼ teaspoon salt
¼ teaspoon pepper
1 cup frozen, mixed vegetables (5 ounces)
⅔ cup rice flour
½ cup potato starch flour
2 tablespoons tapioca flour
4 teaspoons baking powder
2 teaspoons dried parsley, crushed
½ teaspoon dried basil or thyme, crushed
2 large eggs, slightly beaten
¼ cup milk or milk substitute

Directions

1. In a large saucepan or Dutch oven, combine the pieces of chicken, poultry seasoning, salt, pepper, and mixed vegetables with enough water to cover. Bring to a boil. Reduce heat, cover, and simmer for 1½ hours. Remove chicken.
2. Meanwhile, prepare dumplings. In a medium-sized bowl, combine the rice flour, potato starch flour, tapioca flour, baking powder, dried parsley, and dried basil or thyme. Stir in the beaten egg and milk. Set aside.
3. Remove chicken from bones when cool enough to handle. Discard the bones. Cut the chicken meat into bite-sized pieces and return to pan.
4. Drop the dumpling dough by tablespoonfuls into the hot stew. Cover and cook for 12 minutes or until a toothpick inserted in the center of a dumpling comes out clean. Do not remove the cover for the first 12 minutes.
5. Remove the dumplings from the broth into a serving dish. (If left in the broth too long, they become soggy.) Spoon the stew and broth into bowls and add dumplings to bowls.

Makes 6 servings.

Chicken Noodle Soup

Ingredients

3½ cups chicken broth (2 14½-ounce cans)
½ teaspoon dried basil, crushed
½ teaspoon oregano, crushed
½ teaspoon poultry seasoning
1 bay leaf
1 cup broken (1-inch pieces) gluten-free spaghetti
    or fettuccini noodles (4 ounces)
1 cup cooked, diced chicken (½ of a large boned breast
    or 12½-ounce can chunk white chicken, drained)

Directions

1. In a large saucepan or Dutch oven, combine broth, basil, oregano, poultry seasoning, and bay leaf. Bring to a boil. Reduce heat. Add noodles, cover and cook for 6-8 minutes or until the noodles are soft.
2. Discard bay leaf.
3. Stir in chicken and cook until chicken is heated through.

Makes 4 main-dish servings.

Chicken Vegetable Soup: Prepare as above adding 1 cup (5-ounce package) mixed vegetables with the noodles. Continue as above.

Chicken and Rice Soup: Prepare as above substituting 2 cups cooked long-grain rice for the noodles. Continue as above.

Cream of Chicken Soup

Most commercial soups are thickened with wheat flour.
Use this soup for a meal or for a base in casseroles.

Ingredients

2 tablespoons margarine or butter
3 tablespoons potato starch flour (or corn starch)
3½ cups chicken broth (2 14½- ounce cans)
1 cup light cream, milk, or nondairy creamer
2 cups finely chopped, cooked chicken (1 large boned breast)

Directions

1. Melt the margarine in a large saucepan. Stir in the potato starch flour and a dash of pepper, if desired.
2. Add chicken broth and light cream. Cook on moderate to low heat and stir until bubbly, then cook for one minute more.
3. Stir in the chicken and heat through.

Makes 4 main dish servings.

Note: If you use this soup in place of canned condensed soup for casseroles, you may need to allow it to thicken more.

Cream of Potato Soup

Ingredients

1 cup celery, chopped (2 stalks)

½ cup chopped onion (1 medium)

⅓ cup margarine or butter

6 cups potatoes, peeled and diced (1 pound)

2 teaspoons gluten-free vegetable bouillon (2 cubes)

¼ teaspoon pepper

¼ teaspoon dried dill weed, crushed or 1 teaspoon snipped dill weed
   (optional)

1 teaspoon dried parsley, crushed

1 to 1½ cups milk or milk substitute

Directions

1. In a large saucepan or Dutch oven, combine celery, onion, and margarine. Sauté until the onion is tender but not browned.
2. Add potatoes, vegetable bouillon, and 2 cups of water. Heat on high to boiling. Cover and reduce heat. Cook for 15 minutes or until the potatoes are tender. Remove from heat.
3. Mash potato mixture gently with a hand-held mixer or blend in a blender. (Some lumps of potato should be left.) Return to pan.
4. Stir in pepper, dill weed, if used, and parsley. Add milk to desired consistency. Heat to simmering, 5-10 minutes.

Makes 6 servings.

Note: Use this soup in place of canned condensed mushroom soup for casseroles, allowing it to thicken more, if needed.

Serving suggestion: Top with shredded cheese and/or bacon pieces.

Cream of Tomato Soup

Ingredients

2 tablespoons margarine or butter
2 tablespoons sweet rice flour or potato starch flour
1 cup milk
1 14½-ounce can chicken broth
2 15-ounce cans tomato sauce
1 teaspoon dry basil, crushed *(optional)*

Directions

1. Melt the margarine in a large saucepan. Stir in sweet rice flour or potato starch flour and a dash of salt and pepper, if desired.
2. Add milk and chicken broth all at once. Cook over moderately low heat until slightly thickened and bubbly (about 6-8 minutes), then cook one minute more.
3. Stir in tomato sauce and basil, if desired. Cook and stir until heated through.

Makes 4 servings.

Serving suggestion: To dress up your soup, add a tablespoon of sour cream to the center of the bowl and gently swirl with the handle of a soup spoon to form a small spiral. Garnish with a fresh basil leaf or a sprig of fresh dill.

Note: Use this soup in place of canned condensed soup for casseroles, allowing it to thicken more, if needed.

Chili with Beans

Ingredients

1 pound ground beef or turkey
1 cup chopped onion (1 large)
1 or 2 cloves garlic, minced
½ cup chopped green pepper (½ medium)
4 cups tomato sauce (2 15-ounce cans)
2 cups tomato, cut up (16-ounce can)
2 cups kidney beans, drained (16-ounce can)
1 tablespoon chili powder (or to taste)
1 teaspoon dried oregano, crushed
½ teaspoon ground cumin

Directions

1. In a large saucepan or Dutch oven, cook ground beef or turkey, onion, garlic, and green pepper over moderately low heat until meat is browned.
2. Drain fat, if any. Add tomato sauce, tomatoes, kidney beans, chili powder, oregano, and cumin. Stir to combine.
3. Bring to a boil, reduce heat. Cover and simmer for 15-20 minutes.

Makes 6 main dish servings.

Serving suggestion: Top with shredded cheese or sour cream. Serve with hot Corn Bread (page 51).

Winter Soup

This soup freezes well and is convenient to make ahead of time.

Ingredients

1 pound lean ground beef or turkey
½ cup chopped onion (1 medium)
½ cup chopped green pepper
1 clove garlic, crushed
1 16-ounce can tomatoes, cut up
1 8-ounce can tomato sauce
1 10¾-ounce can gluten-free beef consommé (not broth) or
    1⅓ cup water with 1 tablespoon gluten-free beef bouillon
1 tablespoon gluten-free Worcestershire Sauce
½ teaspoon salt
½ teaspoon pepper
⅔ cup red wine (or water)
1 15½-ounce can dark red kidney beans
½ head cabbage, shredded or chopped

Directions

1. In a large saucepan or Dutch oven, sauté ground beef or turkey until brown. Add onion, green pepper, and garlic. Cook on low for 15 minutes or until onion is soft and translucent.
2. Add cut-up tomatoes, tomato sauce, beef consommé, Worcestershire sauce, salt, pepper, red wine, and undrained kidney beans. Bring to a boil.
3. Cover and simmer for one hour.
4. Add cabbage and cook 30 minutes longer. (Soup will thicken when the lid is removed.)

Makes 5 servings.

Serving suggestion: Serve with hot rolls or warm bread. Nothing else is needed for a nutritionally complete meal.

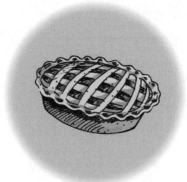

Sweet Treats

Cakes ᛘ Cookies ᛘ Desserts ᛘ Pies

"Why not go out on a limb?

Isn't that where the fruit is?"

—Frank Scully

*"It's a funny thing about life;
if you refuse to accept anything but the best,
you very often get it."*
—Anonymous

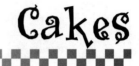

The cake recipes in this section call for one particular size of pan. If you want to bake your treats in a pan of a different size or shape, use the guidelines below for determining baking times.

Pan Size:	Baking times (at 350 degrees)
8-inch round cake pan(s); 1½-2 inches deep	34-42 minutes
9-inch round cake pan(s); 1½-2 inches deep	29-36 minutes
8 x 8-inch or 9 x 9-inch square cake pan(s)	24-36 minutes
13 x 9-inch cake pan	29-36 minutes
15 x 10-inch jelly-roll pan	24-32 minutes
Cupcake pan (half full) {if any of the cups are not filled with batter, fill half-way with water to prevent the pan from warping}	17-24 minutes

If you don not bake frequently, you may not have noticed the new salmonella and bacteria warnings on egg cartons. Eggs should not be left unrefrigerated for more than two hours. The safest way to bring eggs to room temperature before baking is to place them in a bowl of hot tap water for about five minutes.

Busy Day Cake

Ingredients

⅓ cup tapioca flour

⅔ cup rice flour (white, brown, or sweet)

⅓ cup potato starch flour

⅔ cup packed brown sugar

2 teaspoons baking powder

1 teaspoon xanthan gum

2 teaspoons unflavored gelatin

⅓ cup shortening

⅔ cup milk or milk substitute

3 large eggs, room temperature

1 teaspoon vanilla

Directions
Preheat oven to 350 degrees.

1. In a medium-sized bowl, combine tapioca flour, rice flour, potato starch flour, brown sugar, baking powder, xanthan gum, and unflavored gelatin.
2. Add the shortening, milk, eggs, and vanilla.
3. With an electric mixer, beat on low speed until combined, scraping batter down from sides. Beat on medium speed for 1 minute or until well combined. Do not over beat.
4. Pour into one well-greased, rice-floured 9-inch round cake pan. Bake in a 350-degree oven for 29-36 minutes or until a toothpick inserted near the center comes out clean.
5. Cool completely on a wire rack. Invert onto a serving dish and frost, if desired. A nut butter or cream cheese frosting complements this cake nicely.

Makes 6 servings.

Spiced Cake: Add ⅛ teaspoon ground nutmeg and ⅛ teaspoon ground cinnamon *or* ¼ teaspoon allspice with the flours. Continue as above. A lemon-powdered sugar glaze complements this cake. Garnish with lemon rind strips, if desired.

Chocolate Cake: Increase brown sugar to 1 cup and add ¼ cup unsweetened cocoa powder to the flours. Continue as above. A vanilla or fudge frosting complements this cake. Garnish with shaved chocolate, if desired.

Busy Day Pineapple Upside Down Cake:
1. Melt 2 tablespoons of margarine in the 9-inch round cake pan.
2. Sprinkle ⅓ cup packed brown sugar and 1 tablespoon water on the melted margarine.
3. Drain an 8-ounce can of pineapple slices and cut slices in half. (Substitute equal portions of the pineapple juice for the milk, if desired.)
4. Arrange the pineapple slices in the pan (not suitable for cupcakes).
5. Prepare the batter above and spoon on top of the pineapple mixture, being sure to cover all of the fruit.
6. Continue by baking as above, adding 5-10 minutes to complete the baking.
7. Cool for 5 minutes, invert on a serving dish and serve.

Carrot Cake

Ingredients

1 cup rice flour
½ cup tapioca flour
½ cup potato starch flour
2 cups sugar
1 teaspoon baking soda
1 teaspoon baking powder
½ teaspoon xanthan gum
1 teaspoon ground cinnamon
4 eggs
3 cups finely shredded carrot
1 cup cooking oil

Directions   *Preheat oven to 350 degrees.*

1. In a large bowl, combine rice flour, tapioca flour, potato starch flour, sugar, baking soda, baking powder, xanthan gum, and cinnamon.
2. In another bowl, beat the four eggs. Add the shredded carrot and the oil. Mix until well combined. Add to the flour mixture and combine thoroughly.
3. Pour batter into two greased and rice-floured 9-inch round cake pans. Bake at 350 degrees for 60-65 minutes or until toothpick inserted near center of cake comes out clean.
4. Cool on wire racks for 10 minutes. Invert cakes and cool completely before frosting. For traditional carrot cake, frost with sour cream frosting.

Makes eight servings.

Note: If preparing cupcakes, recipe will take longer to cook than ordinary cupcakes.

Classic White Cake

Ingredients

1 cup white rice flour
1 cup potato starch flour
½ cup tapioca flour
2 cups sugar
1 teaspoon baking powder
½ teaspoon baking soda
⅛ teaspoon salt
¾ teaspoon xanthan gum
¼ cup cultured buttermilk powder
1⅓ cup water
½ cup shortening
1½ teaspoons vanilla
4 egg whites

Directions

Preheat oven to 350 degrees.

1. In a large bowl, combine rice flour, potato starch flour, tapioca flour, sugar, baking powder, baking soda, salt, xanthan gum, and buttermilk powder. Add the water, shortening, and vanilla.
2. Beat with electric mixer on low speed for 30 seconds, scraping the bowl occasionally.
3. Add the egg whites and beat on high for two minutes, scraping the bowl occasionally.
4. Pour into two greased and rice-floured 9-inch round baking pans. Bake in a preheated 350-degree oven for 29-36 minutes or until a toothpick inserted near the center comes out clean.
5. Cool cakes on a wire rack for 10 minutes. Cover with another wire rack and invert carefully. Remove the pans. Put the first rack on top and invert again to return the cakes to right side up. Cool completely. Frost as desired.

Makes 12 servings.

Devil's Food Cake

Ingredients

1 cup rice flour, white or brown
½ cup tapioca flour
½ cup potato starch flour
2 cups sugar
½ cup unsweetened cocoa powder
¾ teaspoon xanthan gum
1½ teaspoons baking soda
1½ cups milk or substitute
½ cup shortening
1 teaspoon vanilla
2 eggs

Directions   *Preheat oven to 350 degrees.*

1. In a large bowl, combine rice flour, tapioca flour, potato starch flour, sugar, cocoa powder, xanthan gum, baking soda, and salt. Add milk, shortening, and vanilla.
2. With electric mixer, beat for 30 seconds on low to combine. Beat on high for an additional two minutes.
3. Add eggs and beat on high for two minutes more.
4. Pour into two greased and rice-floured 9-inch round baking pans.
5. Bake in preheated 350-degree oven for 29-36 minutes or until tooth-pick inserted near the center comes out clean.
6. Cool cakes on a wire rack for 10 minutes. Cover with another wire rack and invert carefully. Remove the pans. Put the first rack on top and invert again to return the cakes to right side up. Cool completely. Frost as desired.

Makes 12 servings.

Fudge Brownies

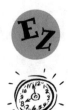

Ingredients

1 cup margarine or butter
2 squares (2 ounces) unsweetened Baker's® chocolate
1 cup sugar
2 eggs
1 teaspoon vanilla
¼ cup rice flour
¼ cup tapioca flour
¼ cup potato starch flour
¼ teaspoon xanthan gum
½ cup chopped nuts *(optional)*

Directions   *Preheat oven to 350 degrees.*

1. In a medium saucepan, combine margarine or butter and chocolate over low heat until melted. Remove from heat.
2. Add sugar, eggs, and vanilla. With a spoon, lightly beat by hand until combined.
3. Stir in rice flour, tapioca flour, potato starch flour, xanthan gum, and chopped nuts, if used.
4. Spread into a well-greased 8 x 8 x 2-inch square baking pan. Bake in 350-degree oven for 30 minutes. Cool on a wire rack.
5. When completely cool, cut into two-inch square bars.

Makes 16 brownies.

Pineapple Upside-Down Cake

This cake takes a little longer to prepare than the Busy Day Cake version, but it is a lighter, fluffier cake, more like the traditional version.

Ingredients

2 tablespoons margarine or butter
⅓ cup brown sugar
1 8-ounce can pineapple slices (reserve juices)
3-4 maraschino cherries, cut in half *(optional)*
¼ cup rice flour
½ cup potato starch flour
¼ cup tapioca flour
1 cup sugar
1½ teaspoons baking powder
½ teaspoon xanthan gum
Milk or substitute
¼ cup shortening
¾ teaspoon vanilla
1 large egg

Directions
Preheat oven to 350 degrees.

1. In a 9-inch round baking pan, heat the margarine or butter in the oven until melted. Remove the pan from oven. Sprinkle the brown sugar evenly over the melted butter.
2. Cut the pineapple slices in half. Arrange the pineapple slices on the brown sugar, all facing the same direction. Place maraschino cherry halves into the holes of the pineapple slices (if used). Set aside.
3. In a large bowl, combine rice flour, potato starch flour, tapioca flour, sugar, baking powder, and xanthan gum.
4. Pour the reserved pineapple juice into a measuring cup and add enough milk to measure ¾ cup.
5. Add the juice mixture, shortening, and vanilla to the flour mixture.

6. Beat with electric mixer on low speed for 30 seconds, scraping the bowl occasionally.
7. Add the egg and beat on high for two minutes, scraping the bowl occasionally.
8. Gently pour the batter into the baking pan, making sure the batter covers all the pineapple slices.
9. Bake in a preheated 350-degree oven for 29-36 minutes or until a toothpick inserted near the center comes out clean.
10. Cool on a wire rack for 10 minutes. Cover with a serving dish and invert carefully (Or serve from the pan and invert the slices onto individual plates.) Serve warm or cool completely.

Makes 6 servings.

Chocolate Sour Cream Frosting

Ingredients

1 cup semi-sweet chocolate pieces
¼ cup margarine or butter
½ cup sour cream (or substitute)
2½-3 cups sifted powdered sugar

Directions

1. Melt chocolate and margarine in pan over low heat, stirring frequently.
2. Cool for five minutes.
3. Stir in sour cream.
4. Add ½ cup powdered sugar at a time, beating with electric mixer until smooth and of spreading consistency.

Makes enough frosting to frost the tops and sides of two 8- or 9-inch cake layers. Store the cake in the refrigerator after frosting.

Microwave Directions

Heat chocolate and margarine in large microwave-safe bowl or in a casserole for 1 to 2 minutes on high power (100%) or until softened. Stir to blend. Continue with step 2.

Sour Cream Frosting

Ingredients

¼ cup butter or margarine
½ cup sour cream (or substitute)
2½-3 cups sifted powdered sugar

Directions

1. Melt margarine in pan over low heat.
2. Cool for three minutes.
3. Stir in sour cream.
4. Add ½ cup powdered sugar at a time, beating with electric mixer until smooth and of spreading consistency.

Makes enough frosting to frost the tops and sides of two 8- or 9-inch cake layers. Store the cake in the refrigerator after frosting.

Microwave Directions

Heat butter or margarine in large microwave-safe bowl or in a casserole for 1 to 2 minutes on high power (100%) or until softened. Stir to blend. Continue with step 2.

Powdered Sugar Glaze

Ingredients

1 cup sifted powdered sugar
¼ teaspoon vanilla
Milk or milk substitute

Directions

1. Place the sifted powdered sugar into a medium-sized bowl.
2. Add the vanilla and 1 tablespoon of milk. Beat with an electric mixer.
3. Add the milk, 1 teaspoon at a time, beating after the additions until the desired consistency is reached.

Makes ½ cup of glaze (enough to drizzle over a 10-inch cake).

Almond glaze: Prepare as above, except omit vanilla and add ¼ teaspoon almond extract with the milk in step 2. Add 1-2 drops yellow food coloring, if desired.

Lemon glaze: Prepare as above, except omit vanilla and add ¼ teaspoon lemon extract with the milk in step 2. Add 1-2 drops yellow food coloring, if desired.

Orange glaze: Prepare as above, except omit vanilla and add ¼ teaspoon orange extract with the milk in step 2. Add 2 drops yellow and 1 drop red food coloring, if desired.

White Frosting

This frosting is firm enough to pipe decorations.

Ingredients

1 cup shortening
2 teaspoons vanilla
4½ cups sifted powdered sugar
Milk or milk substitute

Directions

1. Beat shortening and vanilla together with an electric mixer for 1 minute.
2. Slowly beat in 2 cups of the powdered sugar.
3. Beat in 2 tablespoons milk.
4. Slowly beat in the remaining powdered sugar and enough milk, 1 teaspoon at a time, until the consistency is suitable for spreading.

Makes enough frosting to cover tops and sides of two 8- or 9-inch cake layers.

Variations: Reduce vanilla to 1½ teaspoons and add ½ teaspoon almond extract, lemon extract, or orange extract.

Note: If using food coloring, reduce the amount of milk in step 4 slightly to adjust for the liquid added from the food coloring.

*"We can do no great things;
only small things with great love."*
—Mother Teresa

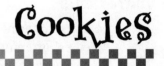

Chocolate Chip Cookies

Toll House cookies like Grandma bakes, only these don't have gluten that will make your child sick!

Ingredients

½ cup margarine or butter (1 stick)
½ cup shortening
¾ cup packed brown sugar
¾ cup sugar
2 eggs
1 teaspoon pure vanilla
2 teaspoons baking powder
2 cups rice flour
¾ cup tapioca flour
½ cup potato starch flour
1 teaspoon xanthan gum
1 teaspoon salt
2 cups (12-oz. package) semi-sweet chocolate pieces
1 cup chopped walnuts, pecans, or hazelnuts *(optional)*

Directions   *Preheat oven to 375 degrees.*

1. In a mixing bowl, beat the shortening and margarine or butter with an electric mixer on medium speed for about 30 seconds.
2. Add the brown sugar, sugar, eggs, vanilla, baking powder, and rice flour. Beat until creamy and thoroughly combined.
3. Beat in the tapioca flour, potato starch flour, xanthan gum, and salt.
4. With a spoon, stir in the chocolate pieces, and, if desired, the chopped nuts.
5. Drop the dough by rounded teaspoonfuls, about 2 inches apart, on an ungreased cookie sheet. Bake in a 375-degree oven for 9 -12 minutes or until the edges are lightly browned. Remove cookies immediately and place on wire rack to cool. Store in a plastic zip-style bag or airtight container.

Makes about 60 2-inch cookies.

Freezer Cookies: Prepare cookie dough as above. Instead of baking the cookies right away, make a dough log about 2 inches in diameter and wrap with plastic wrap. Seal the edges of the plastic wrap and label. Put in the freezer for 2 or more hours. When you want to bake cookies, slice the log into 1/4-1/2 inch slices and bake as above, increasing the time, as needed.

Chocolate Candy Cookies: Prepare the cookie dough as above, except substitute candy-coated milk chocolate candies for the semi-sweet chocolate pieces. (Be sure they are gluten-free.)

Fig Bars

Ingredients

1½ cups dried figs (9 ounces)
¼ cup finely ground pecans or other nuts (4 ounces)
1 cup brown rice flour
1 cup packed brown sugar (7 ounces)
½ cup tapioca flour
¼ cup rice bran
2 teaspoons baking powder
1½ teaspoons xanthan gum
¼ teaspoon salt
½ cup margarine or butter, softened (1 stick)
1 large egg

Directions
Preheat oven to 375 degrees.

1. Place figs in a saucepan. Add enough water to almost cover the figs, about 1 cup. Bring to a boil. Remove from heat. Allow figs to cool in saucepan with water.
2. Meanwhile, in a mixing bowl, combine pecans, brown rice flour, brown sugar, tapioca flour, rice bran, baking powder, xanthan gum, and salt.
3. With a mixer on low, cut in the margarine to the flour mix until crumbly. Add the egg and mix well. Add 2 tablespoons of the reserved fig juice and mix well. Set aside.
4. Put cooled figs in food processor or blender and chop until pasty, like thick preserves. Add 1 tablespoon reserved fig juice at a time, as needed, to get to spreading consistency, but no more than 4 table-spoons. Set aside.
5. In a well-greased 8 x 8 square baking pan, spread one half of the dough evenly. Spread the fig paste, carefully, over the dough. Spread the remaining dough carefully over the figs.
6. Bake in a 375-degree oven for 45-50 minutes or until a toothpick inserted near the center comes out clean and the top is lightly browned. Remove from oven. Cool for at least 10 minutes before slicing.
7. Slice into 2 x 2-inch bars. Remove from pan and allow to cool completely.

Makes 16 fig bars.

Keep refrigerated for up to a week.

Gingerbread Cut-Outs

Ingredients

¾ cup (1½ sticks) margarine or butter
¼ cup molasses
1 cup brown sugar
1 egg
1 tablespoon rice or apple cider vinegar
1 teaspoon xanthan gum
1½ teaspoons salt
1 teaspoon ground cinnamon
1 teaspoon ground ginger
½ teaspoon ground cloves
2½ teaspoons baking powder
1½ cup brown rice flour
1 cup tapioca flour
1 cup potato starch flour
Sugar to sprinkle on top *(optional)*

Directions   *Preheat oven to 375 degrees.*

1. In a large bowl, with an electric mixer on medium to high, beat together margarine or butter, molasses, brown sugar, egg, and vinegar.
2. Add the xanthan gum, salt, cinnamon, ginger, cloves, and baking powder. Beat to combine. Add the flours ½ cup at a time, beating after each addition.
3. Cool dough in the refrigerator for one to three hours or until easy to handle. Divide chilled dough in half.
4. On a lightly rice-floured surface, roll half of the dough to ¼ inch thick. Cut into desired shapes. Place one inch apart on a lightly oiled (or parchment covered) cookie sheet. Sprinkle with sugar, if desired. (If making gingerbread men, use raisins, dried cranberries, or mini M&M® candies, etc. to make the eyes and buttons.)
5. Bake at 375 degrees for 12-15 minutes. Immediately remove cookies to a cooling rack to prevent them from breaking.
6. If desired, decorate with powdered sugar icing or decorative gluten candies.

Makes 40 to 45 three-inch cookies.

Grain-Free Ginger Snaps

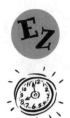

Ingredients

¾ cup (1½ sticks) margarine or butter
¼ cup molasses
1 cup brown sugar
1 egg
1 teaspoon xanthan gum
1½ teaspoons salt
1 teaspoon ground cinnamon
1 teaspoon ground ginger
½ teaspoon ground cloves
2½ teaspoons baking powder
1 cup light bean flour (Garfava, full fat soy, or garbanzo)
1 cup tapioca flour
1 cup potato starch flour
Sugar to sprinkle on top

Directions

Preheat oven to 375 degrees.

1. In a large bowl, with an electric mixer on medium to high, beat together margarine or butter, molasses, brown sugar, and the egg. Add the xanthan gum, salt, cinnamon, ginger, cloves, and baking powder. Beat to combine.
2. Add the flours ½ cup at a time, beating after each addition.
3. On a lightly oiled cookie sheet, drop the dough by measuring teaspoons, 2 inches apart. Sprinkle the cookies with sugar, if desired.
4. Bake at 375 degrees for 12-15 minutes. Immediately remove cookies to a cooling rack to prevent them from breaking.

Makes 150 1-inch cookies.

Variation: Part or all of the light bean flour can be substituted with brown rice flour or rice flour, if desired. Protein levels will be changed.

Freezer Cookies: After mixing the dough, cut a piece of plastic wrap about 18 inches long and lay flat. Place half of the dough on the wrap, shaping it to form a log roll. Roll the plastic around the log roll and smooth the roll with hands. Fold the ends over the log, label, and freeze. Repeat with the other half. To bake, remove log from the freezer, slice in 1-inch pieces. Cut the 1-inch pieces into quarters and roll into balls. Place the balls on a lightly oiled cookie sheet and sprinkle with sugar if desired. Bake as above.

Grain-Free Honey Grahams

Ingredients

¾ cup (1½ sticks) margarine or butter
¼ cup honey
1 cup brown sugar
1 teaspoon xanthan gum
1½ teaspoons salt
1 teaspoon ground cinnamon
2½ teaspoons baking powder
1 teaspoon pure vanilla
1 cup light bean flour (Garfava, full fat soy, or garbanzo)
1 cup tapioca flour
1 cup potato starch flour
¼ cup sugar (if desired)
½ teaspoon ground cinnamon (if desired)

Directions   *Preheat oven to 325 degrees.*

1. In a large bowl, with electric mixer on medium to high, beat together margarine or butter, honey, and brown sugar. Add xanthan gum, salt, cinnamon, baking powder, and vanilla. Beat to combine.
2. Add the flours, ½ cup at a time, beating after each addition. If the dough gets too stiff, add water, 1 teaspoon at a time, until the dough is creamy, yet manageable.
3. Lightly oil a cookie sheet. Scoop the dough, one measuring teaspoon at a time, and lightly pat it on the cookie sheet to about ¼ to ⅛ inch thick. (Use more potato starch flour on your hands if the dough is sticky.)
4. Combine the ¼ cup sugar and the ½ teaspoon ground cinnamon and sprinkle on top of the cookies, if desired.
5. Bake at 325 degrees for 25-30 minutes. Immediately remove crackers to cooling rack to prevent them from breaking.

Makes 90 2-inch crackers.

Variation: Part or all of the light bean flour can be substituted with brown rice flour or rice flour, if desired. Protein levels will be changed.

Chocolate Graham Crackers: Prepare as above, except reduce potato starch flour to ¾ cup and add ¼ cup unsweetened baking cocoa. Omit cinnamon. Sprinkle with granulated sugar before baking, if desired.

Freezer Cookies: After mixing the dough, cut a piece of plastic wrap about 18 inches long and lay flat. Place half of the dough on the wrap, shaping it to form a log roll. Roll the plastic around the log roll and smooth the roll with hands. Tap each side of the log on a flat surface to shape into a long, thin cube, about 2 x 2 inches. Fold the ends over the cubed log, label, and freeze. Repeat with other half. To bake, remove cubed log from the freezer, slice in ¼- to ⅛-inch pieces. Place the slices on a lightly oiled cookie sheet and sprinkle with cinnamon-sugar mixture, if desired. Bake as above.

Grain-Free Nut Butter Cookies

Ingredients

½ cup margarine or butter (1 stick)
½ cup nut butter (peanut, roasted soy, almond, cashew, etc.)
½ cup light bean flour (Garfava, full fat soy, or garbanzo)
½ cup tapioca flour
½ cup potato starch flour
½ cup sugar
½ cup brown sugar, packed (or ¼ cup honey)
½ teaspoon baking soda
½ teaspoon baking powder
1 teaspoon vanilla
1 egg or ¼ cup egg replacer
Sugar to sprinkle *(optional)*

Directions   *Preheat oven to 375 degrees.*

1. In a medium-sized bowl, beat the margarine and the nut butter together until creamy and well combined.
2. In a small bowl, combine the light bean flour, tapioca flour, and potato starch flour.
3. To the first bowl, add half of the combined flours, plus the sugar, brown sugar, baking soda, baking powder, and vanilla. Beat to combine. Add remaining flour and egg. Beat to combine.
4. Scoop out dough, by heaping teaspoons, and roll into balls. Place the balls 2 inches apart on an ungreased cookie sheet. Using a fork, flatten the balls by pressing an "X" into each cookie. Sprinkle with sugar, if desired.
5. Bake at 375 degrees for 11-13 minutes or until the edges are golden brown. Remove cookies to a cooling rack immediately.

Makes 4 dozen cookies.

Variation: Part or all of the light bean flour can be substituted with brown rice flour or rice flour, if desired. Protein levels will be changed.

Lemon Bars

Ingredients

⅓ cup light bean flour (Garfava, full fat soy, or garbanzo)
⅓ cup brown rice flour
⅓ cup tapioca flour
⅓ cup margarine or butter
¼ cup sugar
½ teaspoon xanthan gum
½ teaspoon unflavored gelatin
¾ cup sugar
2 tablespoons tapioca flour
2 teaspoons finely shredded lemon peel
3 tablespoons lemon juice
½ teaspoon baking powder
2 eggs
Powdered sugar (if desired)

Directions   *Preheat oven to 350 degrees.*

1. In a medium-sized bowl, combine bean, tapioca, and brown rice flours, margarine or butter, the ¼ cup of sugar, xanthan gum, and gelatin, beating with an electric mixer until crumbly.
2. Pour crumbs into ungreased 8 x 8 x 2-inch baking pan. Cover with waxed paper. Press down on waxed paper with hands and distribute evenly.
3. Bake in a 350-degree oven for 15 minutes.
4. Meanwhile, in the same bowl, mix the ¾ cup sugar, 2 tablespoons tapioca flour, lemon peel, lemon juice, baking powder, and eggs, beating with an electric mixer on medium speed for 2 minutes or until thoroughly combined.
5. Remove the crust from the oven. Pour the lemon mixture over the hot crust layer. Return to oven.
6. Bake in 350-degree oven for 20 minutes more or until lightly browned around the edges and the center is set. When completely cool, sift powdered sugar on top, if desired. Cut into 2 x 2-inch bars.

Makes 16 bars.

Variation: Part or all of the light bean flour can be substituted with brown rice flour or rice flour, if desired. Protein levels will be changed.

Old Fashioned Sugar Cookies

Ingredients

⅓ cup margarine or butter
⅓ cup shortening
1 cup rice flour
1 teaspoon xanthan gum
1 egg
¾ cup sugar
1 tablespoon milk or substitute
2 teaspoons baking powder
1 teaspoon vanilla
¼ teaspoon salt (scant)
½ cup tapioca flour
½ cup potato starch flour

Directions   *Preheat oven to 375 degrees.*

1. In a large bowl, beat margarine and shortening together until creamy and well combined.
2. Add rice flour, xanthan gum, unflavored gelatin, egg, milk, baking powder, vanilla, and salt. Beat until thoroughly combined.
3. Add tapioca flour and potato starch flour. Beat until thoroughly combined.
4. Cover with plastic wrap and chill three hours.
5. Divide the dough in two. Keep the unused portion of the dough chilled until needed.
6. On a lightly rice-floured surface, roll half of the dough at a time, to ⅛-inch thick. Cut into desired shapes and place on ungreased cookie sheet. (If the dough becomes sticky, return to the refrigerator to chill again.)
7. Bake at 375 degrees for 7-8 minutes (for 2½-inch cookies; less for smaller ones, more for larger ones) or until the edges are firm and bottoms are very lightly browned. Cool on a wire rack. Keep unused dough in the refrigerator until ready to use.

Makes 36-48 cookies.

Pecan Sandies

Ingredients

1 cup butter or margarine
½ cup sugar
1 tablespoon water
1 teaspoon vanilla
1 cup rice flour
⅔ cup potato starch flour
⅓ cup tapioca flour
1 cup chopped pecans (about 2 cups pecan halves)
1 cup sifted powdered sugar

Directions   *Preheat oven to 325 degrees.*

1. In a medium-sized bowl, beat the butter until soft. Gradually add the sugar, beating until light and creamy. Blend in the water and vanilla.
2. In another bowl, combine the rice flour, potato starch flour, tapioca flour, and chopped nuts.
3. Add the flour mixture gradually to the creamed mixture. Mix well between additions.
4. With lightly rice-floured hands, break off small pieces of the dough and shape into elongated balls. Place one inch apart on an ungreased cookie sheet.
5. Bake at 325 degrees for 25-30 minutes or until very light brown. Remove from oven. Let the cookies sit for 10 minutes on the cookie sheet.
6. Roll the cookies in the powdered sugar to coat. Cool completely on a wire rack.

Makes 56 cookies.

Snickerdoodles

Ingredients

½ cup margarine or butter
½ cup potato starch flour
½ cup tapioca flour
1 cup of sugar
1 teaspoon vanilla
½ teaspoon baking soda
½ teaspoon Cream of Tartar
¼ teaspoon ground cinnamon *(optional)*
1 egg
1¼ cups rice flour
2 tablespoons sugar
1 teaspoon cinnamon

Directions
Preheat oven to 375 degrees.

1. Beat the margarine or butter until soft and fluffy.
2. Add potato starch flour, tapioca flour, ½ cup of the sugar, vanilla, baking soda, and Cream of Tartar. Beat to combine. Add the egg, remaining sugar, and rice flour. Beat to combine.
3. In a small shallow bowl, combine the 2 tablespoons of sugar and the ground cinnamon.
4. Roll the cookie dough into one-inch balls and roll in the cinnamon-sugar mix. Place on ungreased cookie sheets two inches apart.
5. Bake at 375 degrees for 11-13 minutes or until the edges are golden. Remove cookies immediately to a wire rack to cool to prevent them from breaking.

Makes about 40 cookies.

*"Change is not merely necessary to life.
It is life."*
—Alvin Toffler

Desserts

Apple Crisp

Ingredients

5 cups cooking apples, peeled, cored, and thinly sliced
¼ cup sugar
2 tablespoons finely ground pecans *(optional)*
¼ cup bean flour (Garfava, full fat soy, or garbanzo)
¼ cup brown rice flour
½ cup brown sugar
¼ cup tapioca flour
2 tablespoons rice bran
½ teaspoon ground cinnamon
¼ cup margarine or butter

Directions   *Preheat oven to 375 degrees.*

1. In a bowl, combine the apples and sugar. Pour into an 8-inch round baking pan.
2. In a bowl, combine pecans, bean flour, brown rice flour, brown sugar, tapioca flour, rice bran, and cinnamon. Cut in the margarine until the crust is crumbly. Pour on top of the apples.
3. Bake at 375 degrees for 30-35 minutes or until apples are tender and crust is golden. Serve with ice cream, if desired.

Makes 6 servings.

Variation: Part or all of the light bean flour can be substituted with brown rice flour or rice flour, if desired. Protein levels will be changed.

Peach Crisp: Prepare as above, substituting 5 cups peeled and sliced fresh peaches for the apples.

Pear Crisp: Prepare as above, substituting 5 cups peeled, cored, and thinly sliced pears for the apples.

Classic Cheesecake

Ingredients

CRUST
¼ cup butter
1 cup finely chopped gluten-free graham crackers (about 25)
½ cup finely chopped walnuts (optional)

CAKE
1 tablespoon unflavored gelatin
2 tablespoons cold water
3 packages (8 ounces each) cream cheese, softened
1 cup sugar
1 teaspoon vanilla
½ teaspoon finely shredded lemon peel *(optional)*
3 eggs

Directions
Preheat oven to 350 degrees.

1. In a small saucepan, melt the butter. Add the graham cracker crumbs and chopped walnuts (if used); mix well. Press crumb mixture onto the bottom of a Springform pan fitted with a flat bottom. Bake for 10 minutes in a 350-degree oven.
2. In a small saucepan, dissolve the gelatin in the water. Heat the combination on low, until it is clear. Set aside.
3. Meanwhile, place the cream cheese in a medium-sized bowl. Beat with a whisk until soft and creamy. Whisk in the sugar and the gelatin mix until well combined. Add the vanilla, lemon peel (if used), and the eggs; whisk until smooth.
4. Pour the batter over the slightly cooled crust.
5. Bake at 350 degrees for 50-55 minutes or until the center is just set. Remove from the oven. Cool 20 minutes on a cooling rack.
6. Carefully run a sharp knife around the edges of the cheesecake. Allow the cheesecake to cool to room temperature.
7. Cover the cheesecake, still in the pan, with foil and refrigerate until it is thoroughly chilled. Then release the side clamp and remove the collar.

Makes 10-12 servings.

Serving suggestion: Top with fresh sliced strawberries, gluten-free cherry pie filling, or chocolate syrup.

Microwave Directions

Place butter in a 1-quart casserole and microwave on high for 45 seconds, or until melted. Continue with step 1. For step 3, heat the gelatin and water in the microwave for 30 seconds or until dissolved and clear. Continue as above.

Creamy Rice Pudding

Ingredients

1 cup rice, uncooked
¾ cup sugar
3 tablespoons cornstarch or potato starch flour
3 cups milk
2 eggs
1 tablespoon butter or margarine
2 tablespoons vanilla
½ cup raisins *(optional)*
Ground nutmeg or cinnamon, as desired

Directions

1. In a two-quart saucepan, combine the rice and 2 cups of water. Bring the rice and water to a boil. Cover, reduce heat, and cook for 20 minutes or until rice is done and the water is absorbed. Remove from heat, set aside.
2. Meanwhile, combine sugar and cornstarch in a heavy saucepan. Add milk and stir. Cook over medium heat until mixture is thickened (6-8 minutes). Remove from heat.
3. In a bowl, beat the eggs. Stir 1 cup hot milk mixture into the beaten eggs. Add back into the milk mixture. Cook until nearly bubbly, but do not boil. Reduce heat. Cook two minutes more. Remove from heat. Add butter and vanilla. Stir gently.
4. Add the cooked rice and raisins, if used. Stir gently.
5. Serve pudding warm with ground nutmeg or cinnamon sprinkled on top or cover the surface of the pudding with plastic wrap and chill for at least 3 hours.

Makes 6-8 servings

Milk-free Rice Pudding: Prepare as above through step 2, except substitute a dairy-free milk for the milk. Stir frequently and cook slightly longer (7-9 minutes) until bubbly and thickened. Prepare step 3 substituting 4 egg yolks for the 2 whole eggs and use a dairy-free margarine instead of butter. Continue as above.

Egg-Free Rice Pudding ⓔz

Ingredients

3 cups milk or milk substitute
½ cup long grain rice, uncooked
1/3 cup sugar
1 tablespoon margarine or butter
1½ teaspoons vanilla
¼ teaspoon nutmeg *(optional)*

Directions

1. In a large saucepan, bring milk, rice, sugar, margarine, and vanilla to a boil. Reduce heat to low, cover and cook 40-45 minutes or until rice is tender and milk is absorbed, stirring occasionally. (It will look like large curd cottage cheese.)
2. To serve warm: spoon pudding into dessert cups and sprinkle with nutmeg, if desired.
3. To serve cold: chill for a least three hours, spoon into dessert cups, and sprinkle with nutmeg, if desired.

Makes 4 servings.

Variation: Add ⅓ cup raisins before boiling, then continue as above.

Creamy Vanilla Pudding

Ingredients

¾ cup sugar
¼ cup cornstarch or potato starch flour
3 cups milk
2 eggs
1 tablespoon butter or margarine
2 teaspoons vanilla

Directions

1. Combine sugar and cornstarch in a heavy saucepan. Add milk and stir. Cook and stir over medium heat until mixture is bubbly and thickened (6-8 minutes). Heat for one minute more. Remove from heat.
2. In a small bowl, beat the eggs. Stir one cup of the hot milk mixture into the beaten eggs. Add back into the milk mixture.
3. Cook mixture until nearly bubbly, stirring constantly. Do not boil (boiling overcooks the egg). Reduce heat. Cook two minutes more. Remove from heat. Add butter and vanilla. Stir gently.
4. Cover the surface of the pudding with plastic wrap. Chill for at least 3 hours.

Makes 6-8 servings

Banana Pudding: Prepare as above through step 3. In a large bowl, thinly slice 2 ripened bananas. Pour the pudding mixture over the bananas. Stir gently. Continue with step 4.

Chocolate Pudding: Prepare as above, except add ¼ cup unsweetened cocoa powder to the sugar, reduce milk to 2⅔ cups, and use 4 egg yolks instead of 2 whole eggs.

Rocky Road Pudding: Prepare Chocolate Pudding. After it is well chilled, add ¼ cup mini chocolate chips and ½ cup mini marshmallows. Stir gently to combine.

Milk-free Vanilla Pudding: Prepare step 1 as above, except substitute a dairy-free milk for the milk. Stir frequently and cook slightly longer (7-9 minutes) until bubbly and thickened. Prepare step 2 as above, except substitute 4 egg yolks for the 2 whole eggs. Prepare step 3 as above, except use a dairy-free margarine for the butter. Continue with step 4 as above.

Milk-free Banana Pudding: Follow the directions for Milk-Free Vanilla Pudding above. Then thinly slice 2 ripened bananas in a large bowl. Pour pudding mixture over bananas. Stir gently. Cover surface of pudding with plastic wrap and chill for at least 3 hours.

Milk-free Chocolate Pudding: Prepare as for Chocolate Pudding above, except follow the directions for Milk-free Vanilla Pudding for the base.

Milk-free Rocky Road Pudding: Prepare as Rocky Road Pudding above, except follow the directions for Milk-free Vanilla Pudding for the base and substitute milk-free chocolate chips (or omit) for the mini chips.

Microwave S'mores

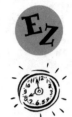

Ingredients

1 rice or corn cake, caramel flavor or plain
¾ ounce of milk chocolate bar (half of a bar)
10-12 mini-marshmallows

Directions

1. On a microwave-safe plate, top the rice cake with the chocolate bar. Then top with the marshmallows.
2. Microwave on 100% power (high) for 18-20 seconds. Let stand for one minute.

Makes one serving.

Variations:

- Substitute the rice cake with Grain-free Honey Grahams (page 222).
- Spread peanut butter or other nut butter over the rice cake before adding the chocolate and marshmallows. Continue as above.
- Replace the milk chocolate bar with two mini YORK Peppermint patties. Continue as above.

Peach Cobbler

Ingredients

8-10 ripened peaches (8 cups, peeled and sliced)
1 cup sugar
2 tablespoons cornstarch
½ cup water
1 cup brown rice flour
⅔ cup potato starch flour
⅓ cup tapioca flour
1 tablespoon baking powder
1 teaspoon baking soda
½ teaspoon xanthan gum
½ cup sugar
1 teaspoon ground cinnamon (optional)
½ teaspoon salt
⅓ cup shortening
⅔ cup milk or milk substitute

Directions

Preheat oven to 400 degrees.

1. In a large saucepan, combine the sliced peaches, sugar, cornstarch, and water. Cook and stir until thickened and bubbly. Remove from heat. Cover to keep hot.
2. Meanwhile, in a medium-sized bowl, combine the brown rice flour, potato starch flour, tapioca flour, baking powder, baking soda, xanthan gum, sugar, ground cinnamon (if used), and salt. Add shortening and mix until crumbly.
3. Make a well in the dry ingredients by pushing to the sides of the bowl with a spoon; add the milk all at once. Mix until completely moistened, but do not over mix.
4. Transfer hot fruit filling to an 11 x 7-inch baking pan. Drop topping dough into 12-15 mounds on top of the hot filling.
5. Bake at 400 degrees for 25-30 minutes or until a toothpick inserted in the topping near the center comes out clean. Serve warm with ice cream, if desired.

Makes 12 servings.

Mock Whipping Cream

A dairy-free alternative to whipping cream.

Ingredients

¼ cup liquid nondairy creamer (like Mocha Mix)
1½ teaspoons sugar
1½ teaspoons egg replacer (Ener-G Foods)
¼ teaspoon vanilla

Directions

1. In a small bowl, combine nondairy creamer, sugar, egg replacer, and vanilla. With an electric mixer, beat on high speed until small peaks form.
2. Use immediately or place in an airtight container and freeze.
3. When ready to use, defrost slightly on countertop and beat again before serving.

Makes 4-6 servings.

Tasty Peanut Butter Balls

Ingredients

½ cup peanut butter or other nut butter (4 ounces)
½ cup honey (4 ounces)
½ cup sweetened cocoa or carob powder (2 ounces)*
1 cup chopped peanuts or other nut (5⅓ ounces)
½ cup sunflower seeds (2⅔ ounces)
½ cup sweetened, shredded coconut (1 ounce)
Powdered sugar to coat

Directions

1. In a mixing bowl, combine peanut butter, honey, and sweetened cocoa or carob powder.
2. Add chopped peanuts, sunflower seeds, and shredded coconut. Stir to combine.
3. Scoop out mixture with small cookie scoop or teaspoon. Roll into balls and dust with powdered sugar (to prevent sticking).

Makes about 60 1-inch balls.

Variation: Substitute chocolate or carob chips for either peanuts or sunflower seeds.

---

* Or use a chocolate-flavored protein drink mix such as GeniSoy® Chocolate Protein Shake.

*"Those who bring sunshine to the lives of others
cannot keep it from themselves."*
—James Matthew Barrie

Pies

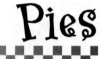

Banana Cream Pie

Ingredients

Single piecrust, baked (page 246)
¾ cup sugar
¼ cup cornstarch or potato starch
3 cups milk or substitute
4 eggs, yolks and whites separated
1 tablespoon margarine or butter
2 teaspoons vanilla
3 medium-sized, ripened bananas
¼ teaspoons salt
½ cup sugar

Directions

1. Prepare piecrust. Set aside.
2. In a medium saucepan, combine sugar and cornstarch or potato starch. With a spoon, stir in the milk until smooth. Cook over medium-high heat, stirring constantly, until mixture is thickened and begins to boil (6-8 minutes). Reduce heat, simmer, and stir for one minute more. Remove immediately from heat and set aside.
3. Set aside the egg whites to bring to room temperature.
4. Preheat oven to 400 degrees.
5. In a small bowl, beat egg yolks with a fork. Add one cup of the hot milk mixture and beat lightly. Slowly pour the egg mixture into the saucepan, stirring rapidly to prevent lumping. Cook over low heat, stirring constantly until very thick (do not boil), about two minutes.
6. Remove from heat. Stir in margarine or butter and vanilla.
7. Thinly slice bananas and place on the bottom of the baked piecrust. Pour warm filling over banana slices.
8. In a medium-sized bowl, beat egg whites and salt at high speed until soft peaks form. Sprinkle in sugar, 2 tablespoons at a time, beating on high speed after each addition until the sugar is dissolved. (Rub a bit

of the meringue between your fingers. The sugar is dissolved when it no longer feels grainy.) The whites should stand in stiff, glossy peaks.

9. With a spoon, spread the meringue over the filling. With the back of the spoon, seal the meringue to the edge of the piecrust to prevent shrinking. Using the back of the spoon, swirl up peaks in the meringue to make an attractive top.

10. Bake at 400 degrees for 10 minutes or until golden.

11. Cover and chill about 4 hours before serving.

Makes 8 servings.

Crumb Topped Apple Pie

Ingredients

PIE:
6-8 cooking apples, peeled, cored, and thinly sliced (6 cups)
¾ cup sugar
2 tablespoons potato starch flour or cornstarch
1 teaspoon lemon juice
Single piecrust, unbaked (page 246)
1 teaspoon ground cinnamon

CRUMB TOPPING:
½ cup brown sugar
¼ cup sweet rice flour (or rice flour)
¼ cup potato starch flour
2 tablespoons margarine or butter

Directions   *Preheat oven to 375 degrees.*

1. In a large bowl, toss the apples, sugar, and potato starch flour together. Sprinkle with lemon juice and toss again. Cover with plastic wrap and refrigerate until ready to use.
2. Prepare the piecrust.
3. Drain the apples and sprinkle with cinnamon. Mix well. Spoon gently into the piecrust.
4. In a bowl, combine brown sugar, sweet rice flour, potato starch flour, and margarine until the mixture is crumbly. Sprinkle on top of the apples. Cover the edges of the piecrust with foil.
5. Bake at 375 degrees for 25 minutes. Remove foil. Bake 20-25 minutes more or until the top is golden and the apples are tender.
6. Drizzle with powdered sugar icing, if desired.

Makes 8 servings.

Pecan Pie

Ingredients

Single piecrust (page 246)
3 eggs
1 cup corn syrup
⅔ cup sugar
⅓ cup margarine or butter, melted
1 teaspoon vanilla
1½ cups shelled, pecan halves

Directions   *Preheat oven to 450 degrees.*

1. Prepare piecrust according to directions.
2. Cover the piecrust with two layers of foil. Bake for 5 minutes in a 450-degree oven.
3. Remove the piecrust from oven and remove foil.
4. Reduce the oven temperature to 375 degrees.
5. In a bowl, combine the eggs, corn syrup, sugar, melted margarine, and vanilla with an electric hand mixer on low or with a fork. Add the pecans, stirring to combine.
6. Cover the edges of the piecrust with foil. Place the pie pan on the center oven rack. Pour in the filling carefully. Bake at 375 degrees for 25 minutes.
7. Remove the foil. Bake 45-50 minutes more or until a knife inserted near the center comes out clean.
8. Cool pie completely on a wire rack. Store in refrigerator.

Makes 8 servings.

Single Crust Pastry

■■■■■■■■■■■■■■■■■■

For a light, crispy piecrust, be careful not to overwork the dough.
The piecrusts do not freeze well.

Ingredients

½ cup rice flour
½ cup tapioca flour
¼ cup potato starch flour
2 teaspoons xanthan gum
¼ teaspoon salt
½ teaspoon sugar
⅓ cup shortening or margarine
4-5 tablespoons ice cold water

Directions

1. In a bowl, combine rice flour, tapioca flour, potato starch flour, xanthan gum, salt, and sugar.
2. Cut in shortening with pastry blender or two butter knives until the crumbs are the size of small peas.
3. Sprinkle 1 tablespoon water over part of the mixture and toss gently with a fork. Push to the side of the bowl. Repeat until all the dough is moistened. Form into a ball.
4. Transfer piecrust to pan using one of these two methods:

   For best results: Place ball of dough into pie pan and cover with plastic wrap. Press dough into the pan evenly from the center to the edges. Press up on the dough to form the crust's edge. Flute the edge while covered with plastic wrap. Remove plastic wrap and fill according to pie recipe.

   Traditional preparation: On a lightly potato-starch floured piece of parchment paper, flatten the dough with your hands. Then roll dough, with a heavy, cold rolling pin, from the center to the edges, forming a circle 12 inches in diameter. Carefully roll the crust onto the rolling pin (use the parchment paper for support, then remove), lift to the pie pan, and gently adjust the pastry to cover the pan. Cover the edge with plastic wrap before fluting. Remove plastic wrap and fill according to pie recipe.

Baked Crust: Prick the piecrust several times with a fork. Bake in a 450-degree oven for 12-14 minutes or until golden. Cool on a wire rack. Fill according to recipe.

Traditional Pumpkin Pie

Ingredients

Single piecrust (page 246)
1¾ cups canned pumpkin (16 ounces)
2 eggs
1 teaspoon ground cinnamon
½ teaspoon ground ginger
½ teaspoon ground nutmeg
¼ teaspoon ground allspice
14 ounces canned sweetened condensed milk (not evaporated milk)

Directions   *Preheat oven to 450 degrees.*

1. Prepare piecrust.
2. Cover the piecrust with two layers of foil. Bake for 5 minutes in a 450-degree oven.
3. Remove crust from oven and remove foil.
4. Reduce the oven temperature to 375 degrees.
5. In a bowl, combine the pumpkin, sugar, and eggs with an electric hand mixer on low or with a fork. Add the cinnamon, ginger, nutmeg, allspice, and condensed milk. Beat lightly.
6. Cover the edge of the piecrust with foil. Place the pie pan on the center oven rack. Pour in the filling carefully.
7. Bake at 375 degrees for 25 minutes. Remove the foil. Bake 45-50 minutes more or until a knife inserted near the center comes out clean.
8. Cool completely on a wire rack. Store in refrigerator.

Makes 8 servings.

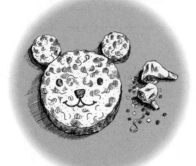

Party & Entertaining Tips

"You don't have to cook fancy

or complicated masterpieces—

just good food from fresh ingredients."

—Julia Child

Menu Ideas for Parties

Plan A

Appetizers
Cubed Cheddar and Mozzarella Cheeses
Cubed Deli Ham or Bologna (check ingredients for gluten)
Potato or Corn Chips

Entrée
Chicken Nuggets (page 135) or Corn Dogs (page 115)

Side Dishes
Baked French Fries (page 182)
Easy Baked Beans (page 188)

Beverage
Fruitful Party Punch (page 255) or Juicy Kool-Aid® (page 39)

Dessert
Birthday Cake or Decorate Your Own Cupcakes

Directions
Prepare the Chicken Nuggets or Corn Dogs ahead of time. Reheat in the oven after removing the Baked French Fries (or keep warm in the oven, but turn the heat down to 170 degrees).

To decorate the cupcakes, place some frosting in paper cups for each color and/or child. Use disposable knives for frosting. Have a variety of cake decorating sprinkles, gummy bears or worms, marshmallows, raisins, candy-coated chocolate pieces, or whatever. Expect a mess, but the kids will enjoy it.

Plan B

Appetizer
Nachos (page 41)

Entrée
Tacos (or Make-Your-Own Taco Bar) (page 131)

Side dishes
Refried Beans (check labels for gluten)
Corn Chips

Beverage
Sport Drink (page 44) or Juicy Kool-Aid® (page 39)

Dessert
Birthday Cake or Snickerdoodles (page 228)

Directions

Prepare as much as possible ahead of time. For a Taco Bar, place each ingredient in a bowl with a spoon to serve with. Topping ideas include shredded cheddar cheese, diced tomatoes, shredded lettuce, sliced olives, sour cream, chopped chives, etc.

Serve the beans plain and allow the party goers to sprinkle the cheddar cheese on, if desired or allowed.

For children with milk allergies/intolerances have some mild salsa or guacamole as a dip with plain corn chips. For easy guacamole, mash a ripened avocado in a small bowl. Add a dash of lemon, a dash of garlic powder, and some drained mild salsa, to taste. Mix well and chill.

Plain corn chips are almost always gluten-free. When flavors are added to the product, the concern for gluten-containing ingredients increases, e.g., Nacho Flavored Doritos® use wheat in the flavoring. Most taco shells will be gluten-free. However, Taco Bell® brand taco products have wheat in them, even the corn taco shells. Check the labels each time you purchase pre-packaged foods.

Plan C

Appetizers

Popcorn (page 43)
Fruit Platter

Entrée

Hot dog slices in ketchup or Little Smokies in Barbeque Sauce (page 111)

Side Dish

Baked Macaroni-N-Cheese (page 156)

Beverage

Fruitful Party Punch (page 255)

Dessert

Decorate Your Own Old Fashioned Sugar Cookies (page 226) or Birthday Cake

Directions

This party menu is not appropriate for toddlers. Popcorn, apples, Little Smokies, and hot dogs are choking hazards for small children who have not mastered chewing effectively. Use common sense and caution when serving these items to children under school age.

Prepare the sugar cookies the day before the party. If you prepare them too far in advance, they will absorb moisture and will not be as crispy. Decorate using the frosting tips for cupcakes in Plan A above.

Prepare the Macaroni-N-Cheese ahead of time, but wait to bake it until 30 to 45 minutes before serving.

Plan D

Appetizer
Buggy Bananas (page 35)

Entrée
Porcupine Meatballs (page 122)

Side Dish
Apple Salad (page 170) or Applesauce

Bread
Dinner Rolls (Rice Tapioca Bread) (page 69)

Beverage
Juicy Kool-Aid® (page 39) or Fruitful Party Punch (page 255)

Dessert
Birthday Cake and Ice Cream

Directions
Prepare the Porcupine Meatballs ahead of time or cook 6-8 hours in a crock pot. The rolls can be prepared the day before and warmed before serving.

The Buggy Bananas are not only a yummy appetizer, but a food craft as well.

Plan E

Appetizers
Ladybugs (page 40)
Baked Potato Skins (page 34)

Entrée
Mini Pizzas (page 146) or Chicken Biscuit Surprise (page 134) or Finger Sandwiches

Side Dish
Creamy Coleslaw (page 171) or Creamy Pasta Salad (page 172)

Beverage
Sport Drink (page 44) or Juicy Kool-Aid® (page 39)

Dessert
Birthday cake

Directions

The Baked Potato Skins can be prepared so that they come out of the oven as the first guests are coming, or you can keep them warm in the oven at 170 degrees for up to 30 minutes.

Mini Pizzas and Chicken Biscuit Surprise can be prepared the morning of the party, without baking, and stored in the refrigerator until time to bake, about 30 minutes before serving.

The Creamy Coleslaw and the Creamy Pasta Salad are better if prepared a day ahead to allow the flavor to develop.

The Lady Bugs are not only a yummy appetizer, but a food craft as well.

Fruitful Party Punch

Ingredients

> 7 cups pineapple juice (2 29-ounce cans)
> 2¾ cups orange juice concentrate (10-ounce can plus 12-ounce can)
> 2 liters ginger ale
> 1 package unsweetened Kool-Aid® Tropical Punch mix

Directions

1. In a large punch bowl, combine the pineapple juice, orange juice concentrate, ginger ale, Kool-Aid® punch mix, and 1 gallon of water.
2. Add 1 party bag of ice before serving.

Makes 34 8-ounce servings.

Attending a Peer's Birthday Party

You can prepare in advance for the times that your child will be invited to a party where gluten-containing foods will be served. Select a cake recipe that your child really likes, such as Devil's Food Cake, and prepare cupcakes. You and your child can frost and decorate these cupcakes. (This is a good time to role-play how your child could respond to questions about his diet that he may be asked at someone else's birthday celebration.)

Place the decorated cakes in an airtight container and freeze. Once the cupcakes are frozen, put individual cupcakes in zip-style freezer bags, labeled and dated, and return them to the freezer. Store the cupcakes in the freezer of your refrigerator for three months or in a deep freeze for six months.

When your child is invited to a party, simply pull a cupcake (or two) out of the freezer and allow the cupcake to thaw on the countertop for one hour.

You may want to send a few cupcakes to your child's school to keep in the freezer for an unannounced birthday celebration or party. The cupcakes can also be put in your child's lunches for school, or for a special treat if not used before the discard dates.

Birthday Cake Decorating

Try your hand at cake-decorating for your child's birthday party! The next few pages will give you a few ideas and get you started.

Teddy Bear Cake

Select a cake recipe (pages 203-207). Prepare cake recipe according to recipe directions except pour batter into baking pans as follows.

For a single-layer cake:

1. Bake in one round cake pan and make two cupcakes for the ears.
2. After baking, cool on a wire rack for 10 minutes.
3. Cover round cake pan with another wire rack and invert carefully. Remove the pan. Put the first rack on top and invert again, onto a parchment paper-covered serving platter, to return the cake to the right side up.

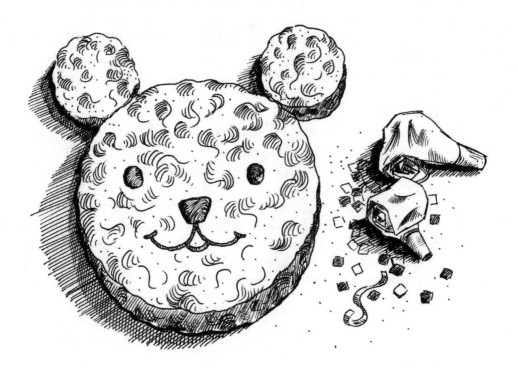

4. Remove cupcakes from pan and cool, right-side up on wire rack.
5. Cool cake and cupcakes completely.
6. Frost main cake with a light chocolate or other light-colored frosting.

7. Position the cupcakes in position for the ears, "gluing" them into place with additional frosting. Frost the "ears" completely.
8. With a serrated knife, smooth frosting in swirl patterns to create "fur."
9. Use raisins, chocolate chips, or piped frosting for the eyes. For the nose, cut a piece of a fruit roll, jellied candy, or chocolate bar, or use piped frosting. For the mouth, pipe frosting to desired expression.

For a double-layer cake:

1. Bake two round layers and 4 cupcakes for ears.
2. After baking, cool on a wire rack for 10 minutes.
3. Cover one round cake pan with another wire rack and invert carefully. Remove the pan. Put the first rack on top and invert again, onto a parchment paper-covered serving platter, to return the cake to the right side up.
4. Cover the other cake pan with the wire rack and invert carefully. Remove the pan. Put the first rack on top and invert again to return the cake to the right side up, on the wire rack (remove top wire rack).
5. Remove cupcakes from pan and cool, right-side up on wire rack.
6. Cool cakes and cupcakes completely.
7. Frost lower layer of cake with a light chocolate or other light-colored frosting on the top.
8. Carefully slide the cake from the wire to the top of the frosted lower layer.
9. Frost top and sides of the cake.
10. Position the lower cupcakes in position for the ears, "gluing" them into place with additional frosting. Frost the tops. Invert the remaining cupcakes onto the frosted lower cupcakes. Frost the tops and sides of the "ears" completely.
11. With a serrated knife, smooth frosting in swirl patterns to create a "fur" look. Use raisins, chocolate chips, candy-coated chocolate pieces, or piped frosting for the eyes. For the nose, cut a piece of a fruit roll, jellied candy, or a chocolate bar, or use piped frosting. For the mouth, pipe frosting to desired expression.

Raccoon Cake

By making simple changes to the previous recipe, you can produce a variety of different animal cakes. To make a Raccoon Cake, prepare the Teddy Bear cake as above using a lighter-colored frosting (Sour Cream Frosting, page 212 or White Frosting, page 214). Using gluten-free chocolate cake sprinkles, create the "mask" of the raccoon. Add the facial features as listed in the Teddy Bear Cake (page 258).

With a little imagination, many different cake themes can be created. A panda bear could have chocolate cake sprinkles on the ears and around the eyes on a white background. Mickey Mouse could be created with dark sprinkles on the ears and the top portion of the head and a large smile. A pig could be created by adding another cupcake for a snout and tinting the frosting pink. The variations are only limited by your imagination—have fun, it's a party!

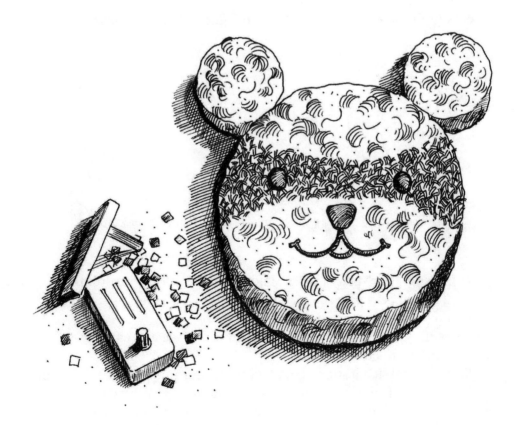

Bunny Rabbit Cake

Directions

1. Select a cake recipe (pages 203-207). Prepare cake recipe according to recipe directions, using two round baking pans.
2. After baking, cool cakes on a wire rack for 10 minutes.
3. Cover one round cake pan with another wire rack and invert carefully. Remove the pan. Put the first rack on top and invert again, onto a parchment paper-covered serving platter, to return the cake to the right side up (piece A, Figure 1).
4. Cover the other cake pan with the wire rack and invert carefully. Remove the pan. Put the first rack on top and invert again to return the cake to the right side up, on the wire rack (remove top wire rack).
5. Cool cakes completely.
6. Cut the second cake according to Figure 1 below for parts B & C.

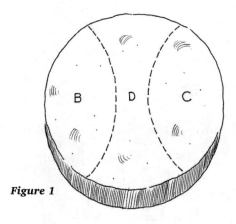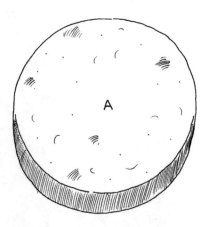

Figure 1

7. Arrange "ear" pieces B & C, and "bow tie" piece D according to Figure 2 on the next page.
8. Frost cake on top and sides.
9. With a serrated knife, smooth frosting on face and ears in swirl patterns to create "fur."
10. For facial decorations (see Figure 3), use raisins, chocolate chips, or piped frosting for the eyes. For the nose, cut a piece of a fruit roll, jellied candy, or chocolate bar, or use piped frosting. For the mouth, pipe frosting to desired expression. Cut a mini-marshmal-

low almost in half, butterfly open and position cut side down, for the teeth.

11. For the bow tie, use a tinted frosting or use same frosting as the face but decorate with candy sprinkles. For the center of the bow, cut a piece of a fruit roll, jellied candy, or chocolate bar, or use piped frosting.

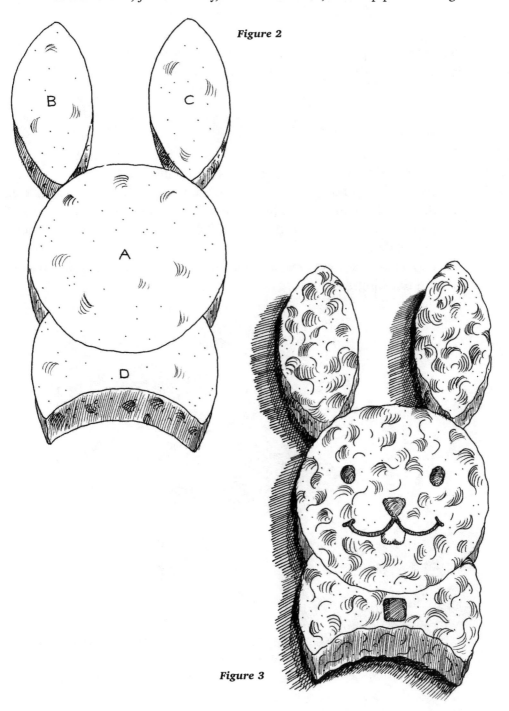

Figure 2

Figure 3

Eight Cake

Select a cake recipe (pages 203-207). Prepare cake recipe according to recipe directions, except pour batter into baking pans as follows.

For a single-layer cake:

1. Bake in two round cake pans.
2. After baking, cool on a wire rack for 10 minutes.
3. Cover one round cake pan with another wire rack and invert carefully. Remove the pan. Put the first rack on top and invert again, onto a parchment paper-covered serving platter, to return the cake to the right side up.
4. Repeat with second cake, positioning it next to the first cake so sides are touching.

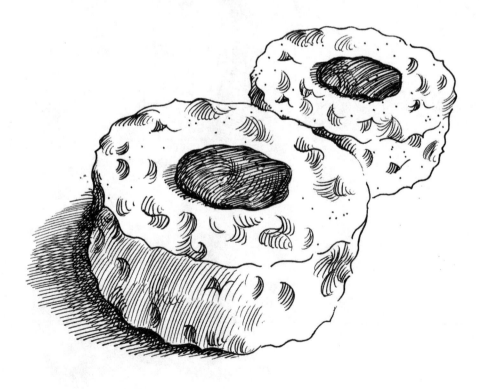

5. Cool cakes completely.
6. Frost cakes.
7. With a serrated knife, smooth frosting in swirl patterns to create texture.
8. With a contrasting colored frosting, pipe a circle in the center of each circle to make the "holes" in the number "8." Pipe writing around the edges of the "8," if desired.

For a double-layer cake:

1. Bake four round layers.
2. After baking, cool cakes on a wire rack for 10 minutes.
3. Cover one round cake pan with another wire rack and invert carefully. Remove the pan. Put the first rack on top and invert again, onto a parchment paper-covered serving platter, to return the cake to the right side up.
4. Repeat with second cake, positioning it next to the first cake so sides are touching.
5. Cover the third cake pan with the wire rack and invert carefully. Remove the pan. Put the first rack on top and invert again to return the cake to the right side up, on the wire rack (remove top wire rack).
6. Repeat with the fourth cake.
7. Cool cakes completely.
8. Frost the two lower layers of cake on the tops only.
9. Carefully slide the third cake from the wire rack to the top of a frosted lower layer.
10. Repeat with the fourth cake.
11. Frost tops and sides of the cakes with the frosting used in step 8.
12. With a contrasting colored frosting, pipe a circle in the center of each circle to make the "holes" in the number "8" and pipe writing around the edges of the "8," if desired.

Baseball Cake

Select a cake recipe (pages 203-207). Prepare cake recipe according to recipe directions, except pour batter into a 1½-quart ovenproof bowl and bake for 55 minutes or until butter knife inserted to the center of the cake comes out clean.

Directions

1. After baking, cool on a wire rack for 10 minutes.
2. Cover the bowl with a parchment covered-serving platter and invert carefully. Remove the bowl.
3. Cool cake completely, at least one hour.
4. Frost cake with Sour Cream Frosting (page 212) or White Frosting (page 214).
5. With a flat knife, smooth frosting, dipping the knife in cool water occasionally, to create a shiny texture.
6. Add red food coloring to several tablespoons of white frosting; stir until color is a dark and uniform red.
7. Use the red frosting to make two rows of "stitches" on the baseball. Place the first row of stitches about one-third of the way from one side of the cake. Pipe a strip of red frosting across the cake from one side to the other. Place the second row of stitches about one-third of the way from the other side of the cake. Pipe short lines of red frosting at right angles to the long stripes of frosting to resemble the stitching on a baseball.

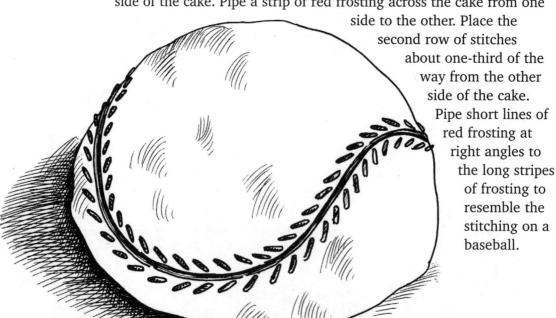

LEGO Cake

Select a cake recipe (pages 203-207). Prepare cake recipe according to recipe directions, except pour batter into 8 mini-muffins (do not use paper liners) and a 13 x 9-inch baking pan.

Directions

1. Bake the cake in baking pan for 29-36 minutes (or until done).
2. After baking, cool on a wire rack for 10 minutes.
3. Cover baking pan with a parchment paper-covered serving platter, invert carefully and remove baking pan.
4. Cool cake completely.
5. Meanwhile, bake muffins for 8-12 minutes (or until done).
6. Cool muffins on a wire rack for 10 minutes.
7. Remove from muffin pan and cool completely on the wire rack.
8. Frost cake with a colored frosting (e.g., blue, red, green, yellow).
9. With a flat knife, smooth frosting, dipping the knife in cool water occasionally, to create a shiny texture.
10. Place the mini-muffins on top of frosted cake, in two rows of four, to resemble the top of a LEGO block.
11. With the same colored frosting, frost the mini-muffins. With a flat knife, smooth frosting to create smooth, shiny texture. Pipe "LEGO" on each mini-muffin in a slightly darker color, if desired.

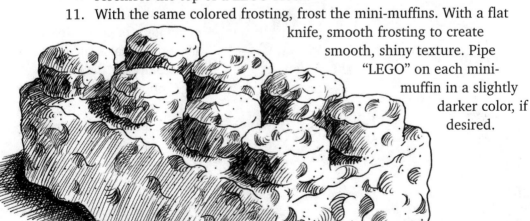

Envelope Cake

This design was created by my daughter, Linda, age 12.

Select a cake recipe (see pages 203-207). Prepare cake recipe according to recipe directions, except pour batter into a 13 x 9-inch baking pan.

Directions

1. Bake the cake for 29-36 minutes (or until done).
2. After baking, cool on a wire rack for 10 minutes.
3. Cover baking pan with a parchment paper-covered serving platter, invert carefully and remove baking pan.
4. Cool cake completely.
5. Frost cake with a light-colored frosting.
6. With a flat knife, smooth frosting, dipping the knife in cool water occasionally, to create a shiny texture.
7. Using a contrasting color, pipe return address (e.g., Mom & Dad) and delivery address (e.g., Child's name, 5th Birthday Party, City and State, etc.).
8. For the stamp, sprinkle colored sugar into a square shape (or cut a piece of fruit roll, or simply use frosting). With a clean, flat spatula, gently press the sprinkles into the frosting. Add a gluten-free cake decoration or cake decorating candy for the design on the stamp, if desired. Pipe the postage price, if desired. Pipe the cancellation lines onto the stamp.

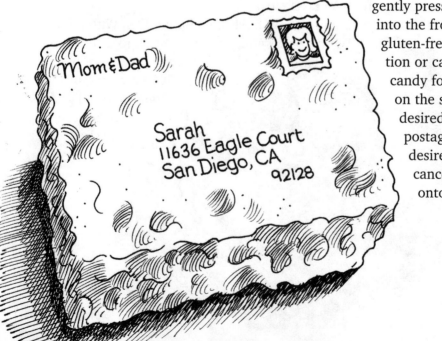

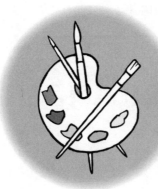

Just for Fun

Craft Recipes

"One of the most obvious facts

about grown-ups to a child

is that they have forgotten

what it is like to be a child."

—Randall Jarrell

Gluten-Free Play Dough

■■■■■■■■■■■■■■■■■■■■■■■■■■■■

Younger children spend a large amount of time learning about their world by touching, tasting, and smelling. Many curriculums have been written to help toddlers and preschoolers explore the world tactilely. One of the major tools used for tactile play in the toddler through kindergarten years is play dough. This gluten-free recipe allows your child to touch, smell, and taste the play dough—if she has to—without harming her health. The unsweetened Kool-Aid® makes for beautiful colors. This dough will last longer stored in the refrigerator, but lasts a long time, either way. If it develops mold or starts to smell bad, it's time to throw it out and make some more.

Ingredients

⅔ cup rice flour
⅓ cup potato starch flour
⅓ cup salt
2 teaspoons xanthan gum
1 tablespoon Cream of Tartar
1 package unsweetened Kool-Aid®, any flavor (or food coloring, but Kool-Aid® is brighter and has a scent)
1 tablespoon vegetable oil
1 cup warm water
Extra potato starch for kneading dough

Directions

1. In a medium-sized saucepan, combine the rice flour, potato starch flour, cornstarch, salt, xanthan gum, Cream of Tarter, and Kool-Aid® powder. (If using food color instead of Kool-Aid®, add the food coloring to the water before adding to the dry ingredients.)
2. Add the oil and the warm water to the flour mixture and mix well.
3. Heat the mixture on medium heat for about one minute or until the mixture thickens and pulls away from the sides of the pan. Remove from heat.
4. Turn out the dough onto a cornstarch-floured board or waxed paper. Knead in enough potato starch until the dough is no longer sticky.

5. Store in an airtight container or zip-style bag when not in use.
6. If the dough becomes too thick or slightly dry after using, heat in the microwave on high for about 30 seconds and knead.

To Dry the Dough into Ornaments: Roll dough out on a lightly potato starch-floured board or waxed paper. Cut out desired shapes. Use a drinking straw to punch out a hole if you want to hang your ornament. Allow ornament to air dry, turning over every 12 hours until completely dried.

Finger Paint

▪▪▪▪▪▪▪▪▪▪▪▪▪▪▪▪▪▪▪▪▪▪▪▪▪

This craft recipe is basic and simple. Margarine tubs make good storage containers. You can also use the empty squeeze bottles that ketchup or mustard come in for storage as well as to control the application of the paint. Remember to always label the contents of anything your child uses for a craft. You wouldn't want the babysitter putting red finger paint on your child's hamburger! Plastic-coated freezer paper makes great finger paint paper, as the coating keeps the paint from soaking through. Commercial finger paint paper is also available.

Ingredients

½ cup cornstarch or potato starch flour
3 tablespoons sugar
2 cups cold water
4-5 colors of food coloring

Directions

1. In a saucepan, combine the cornstarch and sugar. Add the water.
2. Cook over very low heat, stirring constantly until well blended, similar to a thick pudding. Remove from heat.
3. Divide into 4 or 5 portions by pouring into separate bowls. Add 3-4 drops of food color and a pinch of powdered laundry detergent (if desired for easier clean-up) in each portion.
4. Wait until completely cooled before allowing your child to handle the finger paint.

Store any unused portions of finger paint in airtight containers in the refrigerator for up to one week. (Due to the sugar content, which is necessary chemically, it does not keep as well as the play dough.)

Fun Slime

■■■■■■■■■■■■■■ ■■ ■ ■ ■ ■ ■

This type of slimy recipe has been around for years. 20 Mule Team Borax® is the only product I have found that solidifies this recipe. I also recommend the use of Elmer's® School Glue for best results, but other white glues will work okay.

As with any craft recipe, be careful using it on carpet or other porous surfaces. The Fun Slime will stick. Unfortunately, it does not lift off pictures from the comic section in the Sunday paper like the Silly Putty I remember using as a kid. It isn't as bouncy as the commercial counterpart, but it sure is fun to play with.

This is *not* an edible recipe and is not recommended for children who are still putting things in their mouths. If your children make this recipe for themselves, adult supervision is strongly recommended.

Ingredients

1 cup water
6 tablespoons 20 Mule Team Borax®*
½ cup (4-ounce bottle) white school glue
4-8 drops food coloring (as desired)

Directions

1. Pour ½ cup of the water into a small bowl. Add the 20 Mule Team Borax® and stir until dissolved. Set aside.
2. Pour the other ½ cup of water into a medium-sized glass or metal bowl. Add the glue and stir until combined. Add food coloring and stir to achieve the desired color.
3. Pour the Borax mixture into the glue mixture. Knead with hands until most of the water is absorbed and you can form a ball of slime in your hands. Lift the slime from the bowl and discard any water mixture remaining in the bowl. Return the slime to the bowl and allow it to sit, uncovered, for 15-20 minutes or until fairly firm.
4. Store any unused Fun Slime in an airtight container. Keeps for weeks.

---

* To find a retailer that sells 20 Mule Team Borax® in your area, call the Dial Corporation at 1-800-457-8737, or look on the internet at: www.dialcorp.com/storelocator/index.cfm.

Art and Drawing Supplies

For younger children who still put things in their mouths, follow these tips when purchasing art and drawing supplies:

- For crayons made completely from soybeans, try "Prang® Fun Pro" brand. They give awesome color without a lot of pressure required. They are very smooth, but are softer than Crayola® brand crayons and will break easily. Crayola® brand crayons are made from a petroleum-based wax and are gluten-free.

- Most commercially available markers, watercolor paints, and such are gluten-free. Just to be safe, contact the manufacturer before making your purchases if your child may put them in his mouth and you want to be absolutely sure that they contain no glutens.

- Nearly all commercial modeling clay for children contains gluten. Use real clay or prepare the play dough recipe (page 268) to ensure that your child does not accidentally eat bits of gluten-containing clay from under his fingernails, etc.

Easter Egg Dye

Many brands of egg dye are available. Most dyes are gluten-free, but others are not. If you don't plan to eat the eggs, don't worry too much about the dye seeping through the shell. However, if you do plan to eat the eggs, read the ingredient list well or use the following recipe to make your own.

Ingredients

4 teaspoons vinegar per color
¼ teaspoon food coloring per color desired

Directions

1. For each desired color, combine 1 cup hot tap water, vinegar, and food coloring in a large cup or small bowl. Stir gently.
2. Place hardboiled eggs in the cup for 1-3 minutes.
3. Drain eggs in egg carton or on paper towels.

Decorating Ideas

- For two-tone egg colors, hold the egg half-way into the darker color for 2-3 minutes. Remove from first dye and allow to dry. Then place the entire egg into the lighter color for 1-2 minutes. Dry as above.
- To add patterns to the eggs, have your child draw on the egg with a white crayon. Then immerse egg in dye.
- What to do with all those eggs after Easter? Try the Deviled Eggs on page 38 or Egg Salad on page 176.

Appendix: Cooking Tips

"The forest is magnificent,

yet it contains no perfect trees."

—Gye Fram

Baking Substitutions

TO REPLACE:	AMOUNT:	USE:
Broth, beef, chicken	1 cup	■ 1 cup water with 1 cube (or 1 teaspoon granules) gluten-free bouillon
Butter	1 cup	■ 1 cup margarine, or ■ ⅞ cup hydrogenated fat plus ½ teaspoon salt, or ■ ⅞ cup lard plus ½ teaspoon salt
Corn oil	any	■ Any other vegetable oil, such as peanut, sunflower, olive, soy, canola, etc.
Corn starch	1 cup	■ 1 cup potato starch, or ■ 1 cup arrowroot starch
Corn syrup	1 cup	■ 1 cup sugar and ¼ cup additional liquid, or (same liquid as called for in recipe) ■ 1 cup honey, or ■ 1 cup gluten-free rice syrup
Cream, half-and-half	1 cup	■ ⅞ cup milk plus 1½ teaspoons butter or margarine
Cream, heavy	1 cup	■ ¾ cup milk plus ⅓ cup butter or margarine (for use in cooking and baking)
Cream, light	1 cup	■ ¾ cup milk plus 3 tablespoons butter or margarine (for use in cooking and baking)
Egg	1 whole (3 tablespoons)	■ ¼ cup refrigerated egg substitute, or ■ 3 tablespoons pureed fruits or vegetables (like Gerber 1st Foods® or make your own; good choices are applesauce or apple butter, pears, corn, carrots, or mashed potatoes), or ■ 3 tablespoons prepared unflavored gelatin (mix 1 package of unflavored gelatin with 1 cup boiling water until dissolved—keep in the refrigerator and microwave to a liquid before using again) ■ ¼ cup silken tofu, or ■ 1½ packed teaspoons Ener-G Foods' Egg Replacer plus 2 tablespoons water

TO REPLACE:	AMOUNT:	USE:
Garlic	1 clove, small	■ ⅛ teaspoon garlic powder
Herbs, fresh	1 tablespoon, finely chopped	■ 1 teaspoon dried herbs, crushed
Honey	1 cup	■ 1¼ cups sugar plus ¼ cup liquid (same as called for in recipe), or ■ 1 cup corn syrup, or ■ 1 cup gluten-free rice syrup
Mayonnaise (for use in salads and dressings)	1 cup	■ 1 cup sour cream or substitute, or ■ 1 cup cottage cheese, pureed in blender, or ■ 1 cup salad dressing, i.e., Miracle Whip®, or ■ (to reduce fat) ½ cup plain yogurt plus ½ cup mayonnaise
Milk, buttermilk powder	1 cup	■ 1 cup plain yogurt (reduce liquid in recipe by ½ cup), or ■ 1 cup plain soy yogurt (reduce liquid in recipe by ½ cup), or ■ 1 cup liquid milk replacement plus 1 tablespoon lemon juice or vinegar (allow to sit for 5-10 minutes) (reduce liquid in recipe by ½ cup), or ■ 1 cup liquid milk replacement plus 1¾ teaspoon Cream of Tartar (reduce liquid in recipe by ½ cup), or ■ Dry non-dairy milk replacement powder (according to manufacturer's directions to replace 1 cup) plus 1 tablespoon lemon juice or vinegar added to liquid ingredients in recipe, or ■ Dry non-dairy milk replacement powder (according to manufacturer's directions to replace 1 cup) plus 1¾ teaspoon Cream of Tartar
Milk, liquid	1 cup	■ 1 cup non-dairy milk, such as Silken Soy®, Rice Dream®, Westsoy®, Mocha Mix®, almond milk, etc., or ■ For baking, 1 cup fruit juice or potato water (liquid part after boiling potatoes), or ■ 1 cup reconstituted powdered milk replacer, such as Dairy-Free Beverage Mix®, Lacto-free Beverage Mix®, Nutquik®, Soyquik®, non-dairy baby formulas, etc.
Milk, powder	1 cup	■ 1 cup dry powdered milk replacer, such as Dairy-Free Beverage Mix®, Lacto-free Beverage Mix®, Nutquik®, Soyquik®, non-dairy baby formulas, etc. (or amount recommended by manufacturer)

TO REPLACE:	AMOUNT:	USE:
Onion	1 medium	■ 1 tablespoon onion powder, or ■ 4 tablespoons fresh chopped onion
Potato starch flour	1 cup	■ 1 cup rice flour (a denser product will result in baked recipes), or ■ 1 cup corn starch
Rice (3 cups cooked)	1 cup, white, long-grain, uncooked	■ 1 cup uncooked brown rice, or ■ 1 cup uncooked wild rice, or ■ ¾ cup uncooked brown rice plus ¼ cup uncooked wild rice, or ■ 1 cup uncooked converted rice
Shortening, melted	1 cup	■ 1 cup cooking oil (Do not substitute cooking oil for shortening unless the recipe calls for **melted** shortening.)
Shortening, solid	1 cup	■ 1⅛ cups butter or margarine (decrease salt in recipe by ½ teaspoon), or ■ ¾ cup plus 2 tablespoons lard
White sugar	1 cup	■ 1 cup honey (decrease liquid in recipe by ¼ cup), or ■ 1⅓ cup molasses (decrease liquid in recipe by ⅓ cup), or ■ 1 cup corn syrup (decrease liquid in recipe by ¼ cup), or ■ 1 cup firmly packed brown sugar, or ■ 1 cup powdered sugar, or ■ Non-caloric sweetener (follow manufacturer's directions)
Worcestershire sauce	1 teaspoon	■ 1 teaspoon gluten-free bottled steak sauce
Yeast, active dry	1 tablespoon	■ 1 package (¼ ounce) active dry yeast, or ■ 1 cake yeast, compressed

Gluten-Free, Dairy-Free, Egg-Free Baking:
What Went Wrong?

*Information provided by **Jay Berger** of **Miss Roben's,** used with permission.*

Breads

Problem: Breads	Common Causes	Some Recommendations
top browns before inside is done	■ gluten-free baked goods brown prematurely on the outside before fully cooking on the inside ■ soy milk causes darker baked goods ■ oven heat too high	■ cover top loosely with aluminum foil once baked good has achieved desired browning ■ place dough into 2 smaller pans ■ use lighter colored pans ■ reduce oven heat
bottom browns before fully done inside.	■ pan too dark or absorbing too much heat ■ oven rack set too low ■ fat used has low melting point	■ use lighter or glass pan ■ reset oven rack to higher place in oven ■ check type of fat used
still gummy in center, dough very difficult to handle (too tacky)	■ dough too wet ■ not fully cooked inside yet ■ eggs (if allowed) were too large ■ liquids used not at lukewarm temperatures ■ used substitutes that contain extra water ■ not blended well enough ■ too much xanthan gum	■ reduce liquids ■ use liquids at tepid temps ■ check doneness w/flat knife in center ■ check for hidden sources of water (possibly from a substitute) ■ check measurements/tools used ■ divide dough into 2 smaller pans ■ use high power stand-up mixer to blend dough
never rises or loaf too short (unsatisfactory rise)	■ dough too wet ■ not blended well ■ ratio of flour to liquid too low ■ need lighter flour blend ■ too much dough for pan or bread machine to handle ■ yeast stale or killed by too hot liquids ■ too little or wrong egg substitute ■ altitude issues	■ reduce liquids ■ increase ratio of flours/liquids ■ use lighter flour ■ divide into 2 smaller pans ■ blend dough with heavy duty, stand-up mixer before placing in proper capacity bread machine (basic bread setting) ■ use fresh yeast ■ use lighter flour ■ use double baking powder

Problem: Breads	Common Causes	Some Recommendations
never rises or loaf too short (unsatisfactory rise)—ANOTHER POSSIBILITY	■ dough too heavy because not ENOUGH liquids ■ egg replacer and other substitutes used may contain LESS liquid than real eggs and milk ■ substituted flours may be absorbing more liquids ■ very low altitude ■ very humid conditions	■ add more liquid 1 tablespoon at a time until dough correct consistency, blending well in between ■ use less flour ■ if baking at low altitude: increase baking powder or baking soda by ¼ -½ teaspoon, or use dough enhancers (acidic ingredients) ■ decrease liquids ■ decrease oven temperature
rises then falls as cools	■ too wet ■ not fully cooked in center ■ too much dough for pan ■ oven temperature not high enough	■ reduce liquids used ■ check for doneness with flat knife in center ■ reduce oven temperature and bake longer ■ (if in a bread machine) check dough during first knead cycle ■ increase oven temperature
too crumbly	■ dough too dry ■ too much flour-to-liquid ratio (check ingredient measurements) ■ not enough xanthan/guar gum or binding agent (like eggs) ■ water used instead of milk	■ add 1 teaspoon to 1 tablespoon unflavored, unsweetened gelatin, agar (from seaweed), or carrageen (an algae) ■ add more liquid and/or binding agents (e.g., eggs if allowed, or use substitute) ■ increase fat used ■ add milk (if allowed, or use substitute)
dries out & gets stale very fast	■ no preservatives in bread ■ gluten-free goods tend to be more dry ■ not stored properly	■ cool completely, slice, cover well, & freeze unused portions until later (inserting wax paper between slices helps slices pull apart easier later.)
hard to slice	■ not cooled enough yet ■ too dry & crumbly ■ wrong knife	■ let cool completely before slicing ■ see above for dry/crumbly suggestions ■ use sharp, serrated bread knife to slice
as bread cools, gets rock hard	■ dough was too wet ■ too much additional flour used to try to stiffen dough	■ check hidden sources of water and see above tips

Problem: Breads	Common Causes	Some Recommendations
bread very heavy	■ too dense flours used ■ too wet ■ need to blend dough more thoroughly ■ too much flour used ■ not enough leavening agents (yeast, baking powder, baking soda, etc.) used ■ heavy mixer not used	■ reduce amount of original flour used & blend in some lighter flour(s) ■ increase eggs, egg substitute, or baking powder ■ check measuring technique: don't pack down flours when measuring ■ use heavy duty mixer to beat extra air into dough ■ see tips to make dough less wet
bread wet or moist on outside	■ left to cool in pan too long	■ (bread machine) remove from pan per manufacturer or machine directions ■ cool on wire rack
large air pockets in bread or bread "mushrooms" or swells beyond pan edges	■ too much yeast or baking powder used ■ too much egg, egg replacer, or egg substitute used	■ check measurements ■ very high altitudes or hot humid weather accelerates yeast activity—adjust by decreasing liquids some, decreasing egg (or substitute) or baking powder, reduce yeast by ¼ teaspoon ■ when using eggs, be sure each egg measures ¼ cup liquid
dry pockets of dough in loaf	■ not thoroughly blended ■ heavy duty mixer not used ■ dough exceeded bread machine capacity	■ blend thoroughly; ■ use heavy duty mixer only ■ pre-blend before placing in bread machine
rough, rocky surface	■ too little liquid or yeast used ■ too much flour used ■ flour blend used too high in starch ■ exceeds bread machine capacity	■ re-check measurements/recipe ■ try re-blending flours using smaller amounts of starchy flours (potato starch, cornstarch, etc.) ■ check if bread machine capacity can handle dough and amount of dough
bread sticks to pan	■ left to cool too long in pan.	■ remove from pan to cool and place on wire rack

Cookies

Problem: Cookies	Common Causes	Some Recommendations
too soft; undercooked on bottom; soggy	■ undercooked ■ used wrong fat or substitute with too much water content, or too low a melting point ■ too wet ■ too much fat used ■ heat not being dispersed uniformly	■ try cooking longer on lower temperature ■ try more starchy flours ■ try acceptable butter or substitute ■ instead of shortening ■ reduce fat content ■ use darker pan
burns on bottom before done on top	■ oven rack too close to oven bottom ■ dark or non-stick pan used ■ butter used is burning too quickly	■ move rack position up in oven ■ use shiny aluminum pans ■ cookies too thick—spread out dough on cookie sheet with water-damped fingers
too crispy	■ flours used too starchy ■ used butter instead of shortening	■ try some coarser, less starchy flours (rice, corn masa, etc.) ■ try solid shortening or acceptable substitute, instead of butter (and account for extra liquids)
spreads out too thin	■ low-fat, whipped butter, margarine, or substitute used and not suitable for baking, or too high a water content, too low a melting point ■ used oil, butter, or substitute when recipe calls for solid shortening ■ substitute used higher in water content	■ check water content of fat used and recipe directions ■ reduce liquids (especially to account for extra water content in fat substituted—e.g., coconut butter; check package for acceptable substitutes) ■ check fat used (make sure packaging states "good for baking")
falls apart	■ needs more binding agent(s)— such as gums, eggs (if allowed), or egg substitutes (gelatin; flaxseed) ■ not enough liquid used ■ flour to fat-and-liquid ratio too high	■ try an extra egg (if allowed, or use acceptable binding egg substitute) ■ use more xanthan gum ■ use more fat ■ increase liquid-to-flour ratio
cookies too cakelike	■ flour blend used not starchy enough ■ too many eggs (or substitute) ■ too much baking powder used	■ try a more starchy, lighter blend of flours (potato starch, cornstarch, arrowroot) ■ use less egg (or substitute) ■ use less baking powder

Problem: Cookies	Common Causes	Some Recommendations
dough too tacky and difficult to work with (e.g., roll and cut cookies)	■ dough too soft or wet ■ wrong fat used (most common cause) ■ not enough flours ■ needs longer refrigeration	■ check directions for acceptable fats, most roll & cut cookies require solid fats (most common cause) ■ reduce liquids used ■ refrigerate dough or freeze longer before rolling out dough
cookies hard as rocks	■ not enough fat (or acceptable substitute) used ■ dough too wet ■ too much flour added ■ when using egg substitute—sometimes dough still too dry	■ check fat used ■ check amount of flour used ■ account for extra liquids (or lack of them) when substitutions are made
cut-out cookies too tough	■ too much flour used ■ wrong fat used	■ use solid shortening (or substitute) ■ reduce flour on rolling surface ■ start with less liquid and add reserved liquids as needed very slowly
gummy on inside	■ too wet ■ not fully cooked ■ made substitutions and did not account for the extra water in most substitutions ■ cookies too thick	■ check for hidden liquids or additional liquids used ■ reduce oven heat and cook longer ■ make smaller or flatter cookies

Pastas

Problem: Pastas	Common Causes	Some Recommendations
pasta is gummy	■ too little water used ■ overcooked	■ use at least 1½ times the recommended amount of water ■ don't overcook—recheck for doneness every 30 seconds
pasta is mushy	■ overcooked ■ corn pastas tend to be mushier than rice pastas	■ undercook if using in another recipe (e.g., lasagna), or re-heating later ■ try rice pastas
pasta is hard on the inside	■ not cooked long enough	■ check doneness every 30 seconds by tasting until desired texture is reached

Cakes / Muffins / Cupcakes

Problem: Cakes/Muffins/Cupcakes	Common Causes	Some Recommendations
browns prematurely on outside before done on inside	■ pan size too small or pan color too dark ■ inherent nature of gluten-free and soy goods (and some sugar substitutes) ■ oven heat too high	■ adjust oven rack ■ use lighter colored or larger pan, or place batter in 2 smaller pans ■ reduce oven temperature and increase baking time
collapses as cools	■ too wet ■ not fully cooked ■ too much batter for pan	■ check liquids and measurements, and account for extra liquids with substitutions made ■ check for doneness with a flat knife
too crumbly	■ not enough liquid or fat used ■ overcooked	■ check recipe and measurements ■ reduce cooking time ■ add more moisture and/or fat
never rises	■ too heavy ■ too wet ■ oven temperature too low ■ needs more binding agent(s), such as gums, eggs (if allowed), or egg substitutes (gelatin; flaxseed) ■ angel food cake—batter includes traces of fat or wrong pan used	■ try lighter flours ■ use more leavening such as eggs (if allowed) or baking powder ■ ensure egg substitute used provides leavening ■ check oven temperature and baking times ■ check for proper doneness
too heavy or dense	■ flours too coarse ■ not enough liquid or fat ■ milk, fat, or sugar substitute used made batter too wet ■ sugar deleted from recipe but not replaced with an acceptable substitute ■ too much batter for the pan	■ try lighter flours ■ check measurements ■ use acceptable sugar substitute that replaces most of the bulk of the sugar ■ account for extra liquids in substitutes used ■ use extra baking powder or egg substitute ■ split batter into 2 smaller pans
gummy on inside	■ too wet ■ not fully cooked ■ made substitutions and did not account for the extra water in most substitutes ■ cake, cupcake, or muffin tin filled too full	■ check for hidden liquids or additional liquids used ■ reduce oven heat and cook longer ■ use 2 smaller pans ■ reduce oven temperature, cover lightly with aluminum foil, and cook longer ■ check doneness with knife test ■ fill batter only $\frac{1}{2}$ - $\frac{2}{3}$ full

Problem: Cakes/ Muffins/Cupcakes	Common Causes	Some Recommendations
too wet on outside when cooled or stored	■ not properly cooled before frosting or storing ■ stored in too warm or humid a location	■ cool completely before frosting and/or storing and keep in tightly sealed container away from heat
top cracks or splits	■ over-baked ■ too hot an oven temperature ■ with some cakes (e.g., pound cake) this is expected and desired	■ check for doneness with knife test and cover top as needed with aluminum foil ■ reduce oven temperature
too difficult to frost	■ not yet cooled completely ■ not removed properly from pan ■ frosting not of suitable spreading consistency ■ excess crumbs not brushed away ■ frosting a still frozen cake, muffin, or cupcake	■ wait until completely cool (or thawed) before frosting ■ soften frosting consistency (and make sure at room temperature) ■ check pan removal (see below)
difficult to remove from pan	■ pan not greased heavily enough ■ cooled improper amount of time (too little time can cause fragile cake form to break; too much time and cake top can cool and begin to harden to pan edges)	■ loosen cake or muffin edges gently with spatula or thin knife before removal ■ grease pan adequately ■ let cool some before removal
layers or tops uneven	■ oven rack not level ■ pans warped ■ not centered in oven	■ check oven position and racks ■ check that pans are flat
overflows or mushrooms beyond pan edges/top	■ too much batter for pan ■ too much egg or substitute ■ too much baking powder ■ pan filled too high to top of pan	■ use 2 smaller or 1 larger pan ■ reduce egg or substitute ■ reduce baking powder ■ fill pan or forms only $\frac{1}{2}$-$\frac{2}{3}$ full
cupcakes cook unevenly	■ unused/empty cupcake forms in pan, causing uneven heating ■ pan warped ■ not centered in oven ■ cupcake forms not filled even amounts	■ fill unused muffin tins with water to evenly distribute heat to cupcakes ■ center pan in oven ■ check rack position ■ fill each cupcake form equally $\frac{1}{2}$-$\frac{2}{3}$ full

Pancakes, Pizza

Problem: Pancakes, Pizza	Common Causes	Some Recommendations
gummy inside	■ too wet ■ undercooked or cooked unevenly ■ oven temperature too high ■ used substitutes and didn't account for extra liquid ■ liquids used too cold ■ pizza toppings too wet	■ reduce oven/stove heat ■ adjust position of rack in oven ■ use liquids (including eggs or substitutes) at room temperature ■ reduce liquids if using substitutes, especially rice milk
browns prematurely on bottom	■ pan heat or oven temperature too hot or concentrating heat more at bottom ■ pizza shell too thick	■ reduce oven/stove heat ■ cook at lower temperature for longer time ■ account for liquids in toppings/additions ■ try pre-baking pizza some before adding toppings
too heavy	■ flours too heavy ■ too much flour used ■ dough too wet	■ try lighter blend of flours ■ watch measurements ■ check for hidden liquids in substitutes
pizza dough difficult to roll out, too tacky	■ dough too wet ■ did not account for substitutions made ■ not enough flour used ■ did not dust surface prior to handling	■ account for hidden liquids ■ use liquids at room temperature ■ adjust liquids-to-flour ratio ■ account for additional liquids in substitutes
pizza toppings done before dough finished cooking	■ dough formed too thick ■ oven temperature too high ■ rack position in oven too high	■ pre-cook pizza shell some before adding toppings ■ reduce oven temperature and cook longer ■ tent top of pizza lightly with aluminum foil

Metric Equivalents

Weight

1 tablespoon =	3 teaspoons	.5 fluid ounce	14.8 milliliters
1 cup =	16 tablespoons	8 fluid ounces	236.6 milliliters
1 pint=	2 cups	16 fluid ounces	473.2 milliliters
1 quart =	2 pints	32 fluid ounces	946.4 milliliters
1 gallon =	4 quarts	128 fluid ounces	3.78 liters

Volume

U.S.	Metric	U.S.	Metric
¼ ounce	7 grams	½ ounce	14 grams
1 ounce	28 grams	1¼ ounces	35 grams
1½ ounces	40 grams	1⅔ ounces	45 grams
2 ounces	55 grams	2½ ounces	70 grams
4 ounces	112 grams	5 ounces	140 grams
8 ounces	228 grams	10 ounces	280 grams
15 ounces	425 grams	16 ounces (1 pound)	454 grams
¼ cup	60 milliliters	⅓ cup	80 milliliters
½ cup	120 milliliters	⅔ cup	160 milliliters
1 cup	240 milliliters	1¼ cups	300 milliliters
1½ cups	360 milliliters	1⅔ cups	400 milliliters
3 cups	700 milliliters	4 cups (1 quart)	.95 liter
1.06 quarts	1 liter	4 quarts (1 gallon)	3.8 liters

Temperature Conversion Rates

°Fahrenheit	°Celsius	British Gas (Rogulo) Mark	Heat level
120°	49°	N/A	
130°	55°	N/A	
200°	95°	0	Very cool
225°	110°	¼	Very cool
250°	120°	½	Very cool
275°	135°	1	Cool or slow
300°	150°	2	Cool or slow
325°	165°	3	Warm
350°	175°	4	Moderate
375°	190°	5	Moderately hot
400°	200°	6	Fairly hot
425°	220°	7	Hot
450°	230°	8	Very hot
475°	245°	9	Very hot

High Altitude Cooking*

If you are cooking at altitudes over 3,000 feet above sea level, you may need to make changes in time, temperature, or recipes when preparing food. The higher the atmosphere is above sea level, the lower the atmospheric pressure is. Water and other liquids evaporate faster and boil at a lower temperature at decreased atmospheric pressures. In addition, leavening gases in breads and cakes expand more than at sea level. This section will provide some hints for food preparation at various altitudes and for different food preparation techniques.

Stovetop Cooking

The point at which the pressure of water vapor equals the atmospheric pressure is called the boiling point. If the atmospheric pressure is lower, the pressure required to reach the boiling point is also lower. The lower the boiling point, the longer your cooking times will be. The following chart summarizes the boiling temperatures of water at different altitudes.

Approximate Boiling Temperatures of Water at Various Altitudes	
Altitude	Temperature to boiling
Sea level	212 degrees F
2,000 feet	208 degrees F
5,000 feet	203 degrees F
7,500 feet	198 degrees F
10,000 feet	194 degrees F

Deep-fat Frying

At higher altitudes, fats used for frying should not be heated to the same temperature as they are at lower altitudes. Lowering the temperature will prevent food from being overcooked on the outside and undercooked on the inside. The decrease in temperature needed depends on the food being fried, but a good rule of thumb is to lower the frying temperature about 3 degrees Fahrenheit for every increase of 1,000 feet in elevation.

---

* Adapted from information provided in Pamphlet 41, prepared by Pat Kendall, food science and human nutrition specialist and professor, Colorado State University Cooperative Extension.

Puddings and Cream-Pie Fillings

Above 5,000 feet, a double boiler can not reach temperatures high enough to properly cook starches such as those in puddings. It is best to use direct heat (cook ingredients in a saucepan directly above stove burner) to prepare puddings and cream-pie fillings at these altitudes.

Breads

Higher altitudes have a marked effect on the rising time of bread. At high altitudes, the rising times are shorter than at sea level. Since achieving a good flavor in bread products is partially dependent on the length of time the bread rises, it is a good idea to allow the bread to rise the entire recommended time. Stirring gluten-free bread dough once, as in a traditional bread recipe, should allow enough time for the flavor to develop without making the bread too dense.

In addition, flours tend to be drier and able to absorb more fluid in high, dry climates. Less flour may be needed to make the dough the proper consistency than is listed in the recipes.

Cakes Made with Shortening

Most cake recipes will need no modifications when prepared up to 3,000 feet in elevation. Above that, cakes may rise excessively, causing a coarse texture, or cakes may fall. To avoid these problems, decrease the amount of baking powder or soda. Also increase the baking temperature 15 to 25 degrees. This will "set" the batter before the cake expands too much. You may also want to decrease the sugar and add liquids, since water evaporates more quickly, resulting in a higher concentration of sugar in baked goods. Repeated experimentation with each recipe is the only way to discover the most successful proportions to use. The following table provides a starting place. Try the smaller adjustments first, and then work up if needed.

Cake recipe adjustment guide at various altitudes.			
Adjustment	*3,000 feet*	*5,000 feet*	*7,000 feet*
Reduce baking powder. For each teaspoon called for, decrease by:	⅛ teaspoon	⅛–¼ teaspoon	¼ teaspoon
Reduce sugar. For each cup called for, decrease by:	0-1 tablespoon	0-2 tablespoons	1-3 tablespoons
Increase liquid. For each cup called for, add:	1-2 tablespoons	2-4 tablespoons	3-4 tablespoons

Cookies

Many cookie recipes have acceptable results at high altitudes. You may be able to bake better cookies, however, by: slightly increasing baking temperature; slightly decreasing baking powder or soda, fat, and/or sugar; and slightly increasing fluids and flour.

Biscuits, Muffins, and Quick Breads

Quick breads with a cake-like structure usually can be improved at high altitudes by following the adjustment recommendations for cakes.

Quick breads with a muffin-like structure may cook to an acceptable consistency without any adjustments to the recipe. However, sometimes these baked goods may have a bitter or alkaline flavor due to the differences in how baking powder or soda act at higher altitudes. If this occurs, reduce the baking powder or soda slightly the next time you try the recipe.

Pie Crusts

Pie crusts are not generally affected by altitude, but using slightly more fluid may produce better results.

Practical Notes for High Altitude Baking

- Do not assume that your recipe will fail. Try it first. It may need little or no modification.
- Use the same flours you would at sea level. No special brands or equipment are needed.
- For more information on cooking at high altitudes, contact your local county extension office or contact:

> Cooperative Extension
> 1 Administration Building
> Colorado State University
> Fort Collins, CO 80523-4040
> (970) 491-6281
> Fax (970) 491-6208
> www.ext.colostate.edu

Resources

Gluten-Free Suppliers

*"Thousands of candles can be lighted from a single candle,
and the life of the candle will not be shortened.
Happiness never decreases by being shared."*

—Buddha

Adrienne's Gourmet Foods
849 Ward Drive
Santa Barbara, CA 93111
(800) 937-7010; (805) 964-6848 (8 AM to 5 PM PST)
Web Site: www.adriennes.com
Maker of Papadini® Hi-Protein Pure Lentil Bean Pasta available in four cuts, Orzo, Mafalda, Cresta di Gallo, and Conchigliette.

Authentic Foods
1850 West 169th Street, Suite B
Gardena, CA 90247
(800) 806-4737
Web site: www.authenticfoods.com
    Specialty bean flours, rice flours, corn flour, tapioca flour, potato flour, potato starch flour, specialty xanthan gum, specialty vanilla powder, maple sugar, and many baking mixes.

Barry Farm
20086 Mudsock Road
Wapakoneta, OH 45895

(419) 228-4640 (Mon. – Sat., 9 AM–9 PM EST)
Web site: www.barryfarm.com
    Basic gluten-free flours, gluten-free baking mixes, pastas, all kinds of grains, jams, jellies, pickles, relishes, and sauces. All certified organic.

Bob's Red Mill Natural Foods
5209 SE International Way
Milwaukie, OR 97222
(800) 349-2173 (Mon. – Fri., 8 AM–5 PM PST)
FAX: (503) 653-1339
Web site: www.bobsredmill.net
    Sells many gluten-free flours, prepared in a clean room, reducing cross-contamination.

'Cause You're Special
P.O. Box 316
Phillips, WI 54555
(715) 339-6959
FAX: (603) 754-0245
Web site: www.causeyourespecial.com
    Provides wheat-free, gluten-free, all natural products, and gourmet baking mixes.

De-Ro-Ma (1983) Ltée Food Intolerance Centre
1118 Berlier
Lavel, Quebec, Canada H7L 3R9
(800) 363 3438 or (800) 363-DIET
FAX: (450) 629-4781
Web site: www.glutino.com
    Baking mixes, various gluten-free flours, prepared breads, rusks & crackers, soups & sauces, pasta, cookies, sweets & desserts, cereals, frozen products, egg replacers, milk substitutes, baking powder, guar & xanthan gums, yeasts, and some gluten- and sugar-free foods.

Dietary Specialties
P.O. Box 227
Rochester, NY 14601
(716) 263-2787
(800) 544-0099 (Mon. – Fri., 8:30 AM–5:00 PM EST)
    Breads, crackers, cookies, pasta, baking mixes, white rice flour, potato starch flour, tapioca flour, guar & xanthan gums, gluten-free flavor extracts, rice starch, rice crumb, condiments and spices, and snacks.

El Peto Products, LTD
41 Shoemaker Street, Unit 2-3
Kitchener, Ontario, Canada N2E 3G9
(800) 387-4064 (Toll free in U.S. and Canada)
FAX: (519) 748-5279
Web site: www.elpeto.com
    Pastas, baked products, Christmas items, soups & sauces, cereals, crackers, ready-to-use doughs, baking mixes, flours, guar and xanthan gums, and baking powder.

ENER-G Foods
P.O. Box 84487
5960 1st Ave. S.
Seattle, WA 98124-5787
(800) 331-5222; (206) 767-6660
FAX: (206) 764-3398
Web site: www.ener-g.com
     Gluten-free baked products, breads, yeast-free breads, cakes, doughnuts, cookies and snacks, baking mixes, egg replacer, whole egg powder, dry vinegar, Bette Hagman's Gluten-Free Gourmet Blend, Bette Hagman's Four Flour Bean Mix, rice flours, soy flour, tapioca flour, potato starch flour, potato flour, rice bran, rice polish, cultured buttermilk powder, milk-free beverage mixes, xanthan gum, dessert mixes, pastas, soup mixes, cereals, crackers, and specialty order items.

Food-for-Life Baking Co.
Web site: www.food-for-life.com
     Sells gluten-free breads and banana muffins online. Has a search facility to help find a retailer near you.

Foods by George
Web site: www.foodsbygeorge.com
     Gluten-free frozen bakery items (English muffins, pecan tarts, crumb cakes) and pasta products. Initially known for his ravioli.

Gifts of Nature
P.O. Box 309
Corvallis, MT 59828
(406) 961-1529
FAX: (406) 961-3491
Web site: www.giftsofnature.net
     Sells a gluten-free flour blend that is a one-for-one substitution for flour in any recipe. Specializes in baking mixes made with brown rice and bean flours.

Gillian's Foods
55 Centre Street
Lynn, MA 01905
(781) 286-4095
Web site: www.gilliansfoods.com
     Specializes in gluten-free rolls and other bread items. People rave about the dinner rolls.

The Gluten-Free Mall
Web site: www.glutenfreemall.com
     A "one-stop shop" on the Internet for gluten-free and wheat-free products. The Mall combines the complete catalogues of many different gluten-free food companies, but orders are actually placed individually with each company, so shipping costs are increased if you order from more than one vendor.

The Gluten-Free Pantry, Inc.
P.O. Box 840
Glastonbury, CT 06033

(860) 633-3826 (for inquiries; Mon.–Fri. , 9 AM–5 PM, EST)
(800) 291-8386 (orders only)
FAX: (860) 633-6853
Web site: www.glutenfree.com

Gluten-free bread mixes, cake mixes, pie crust mixes, muffin mixes, pancake mixes, cookie mixes, appliances & accessories, yeast, ascorbic acid, cookies, crackers, rice sticks, snacking rings, pretzels, gluten-free vitamins, rice flours, potato starch flour, Jowar flour, tapioca flour, gluten-free flavorings, ground milled flaxseed, lecithin, chocolate chips, chickpea flour, wild red corn meal, xanthan & guar gums, almond flour, powdered egg whites, cheddar cheese powder, cereal, condiments, pastas, exotic rice, and soup mixes.

Gluten Free Trading Co.
604A W. Lincoln Avenue
Milwaukee, WI 53215
(888) 993-9933; (414) 385-9950
FAX: (414) 385-9915
Web site: www.gluten-free.net

Gluten-free and celiac safe groceries from around the world.

Gluten Solutions, Inc.
3810 Riviera Drive, Suite 1
San Diego, CA 92109
(888) 845-8836; (858) 483-8877
Web site: www.glutensolutions.com

Over 235 gluten-free foods, plus an assortment of books and cookware.

Glutino
(800) 363-DIET (3438); (450) 629-7689
Web site: www.glutino.com

A Quebec-based firm with an extensive line of gluten-free products that they import from all around the world, as well as a line of their own products.

Jowar Foods
P.O. Box 775
Vega, TX 79092
(806) 267-0820
FAX: (806) 267-0769
Web site: www.jowar.com

Produces sorghum-based food products, including Jo-Krisps.

King Arthur Flour
P.O. Box 876
Norwich, VT 05055-0876
(800) 827-6836
Web sites: www.kingarthurflour.com
www.BakersCatalogue.com

Their Baker's Catalogue® is very thorough. Most items are *not* gluten-free; however, there are some flours, flavors, yeasts, non-instant non-fat dried milk powder, ketchups that can be used, as well as more things to bake with than can be imagined. "A catalogue of fine tools, ingredients, equipment, and books for the home baker."

Kinnikinnick Foods

10306-112 Street
Edmonton, Alberta, Canada T5K 1N1
(877) 503-4466; (780) 424-2900
FAX: (780) 421-0456
Web site: www.kinnikinnick.com

    Distributes 500 products that are 100 percent gluten-free. Quality controls are so strict that employees may not even bring gluten-containing foods onto the premises.

Lundberg Family Farms

P.O. Box 369
Richvale, CA 95974-0369
(530) 882-4551
FAX: (530) 882-4500
Web site: www.lundberg.com

    Produces rice specialty products.

Miss Roben's

P.O. Box 1149
Frederick, MD 21702
(800) 891-0083; (301) 631-5594
Website: www.missroben.com

    Gluten-free breads and buns, snacks, crackers, cakes, muffins, cookies, cereal, puddings, pizza crust, pie crusts, pastas, candies, side dishes, gluten-free flours, gluten-free mixes, dough enhancers, flavorings, extracts, gums and baking powder, sauces and gravies, soups, bakeware, books and videos, personal care, vitamins. Also has a special service of custom mixes.

Mona's Gluten-Free

1462 Jamaica Road
Victoria, BC, Canada V8N 2C8
Web site: www.madebymona.com

    A company operated by an individual with celiac disease, offering online purchase of gluten-free baking mixes in single units or in bulk. (Some restrictions apply.)

Mrs. Leeper's Pasta

12455 Kerran Street, #200
Poway, CA 92064-6855
(858) 486-1101
FAX: (858) 486-5115
Web site: www.mrsleeperspasta.com

    Produces a line of corn and rice pastas in many shapes.

Nana's Kitchen

P.O. Box 704
527B Lakeshore Drive
Chase, BC, Canada V0E 1M0
(866) 679-2818
Or
P.O. Box 2640
Oroville, WA 98844

(250) 679-2818
FAX: (250) 679-2817
Web site: www.cookingwithnana.com
      Produces a gadget called a Spaetzle Board for making gluten-free pasta. Website recipes for gluten-free pasta.

Pamela Products
335 Allerton Avenue
South San Francisco, CA 94080
(650) 952-4546
FAX: (650) 742-6643
Web site: www.pamelasproducts.com
      Produces a line of gluten-free cookies available in health food stores and online health food stores. Also produces some biscotti and baking mixes.

Quinoa Corporation
P.O. Box 1039
Torrance, CA 90505
(310) 530-8666 (Mon.–Fri., 8 AM–3 PM PST)
Web site: www.quinoa.net
      Makers of Ancient Harvest Brand Quinoa®. Products include: Ancient Harvest Quinoa Flakes, an alternative for oatmeal; Wheat-Free Supergrain Pasta in various shapes, Elbows, Shells, Garden Pagodas, Rotelle, Linguine, Spaghetti, & Veggie Curls; Ancient Harvest Quinoa Flour; and Whole Grain Quinoa.

True Foods Market
1537 South 125 East
Orem, UT 84058
877-274-5914 (Toll free in U.S. and Canada)
(801) 491-3274 (outside U.S. and Canada)
Web site: www.truefoodsmarket.com
      Baking ingredients, seasonings, beverages, books and supplies, cereals, fruits and sweeteners, grains and legumes, housewares, cleaners and tools, nuts and seeds, packaged entrees, personal care, snacks and treats, sprouting supplies, and holiday requests.

Food Manufacturer Resources

> *"Parents are often so busy with the physical rearing of children*
> *that they miss the glory of parenthood,*
> *just as the grandeur of the trees is lost when raking the leaves."*
> —Marcelene Cox

This section is designed to be a quick resource for you to be able to confirm the gluten-free status of your favorite products. Most of the companies listed in this section provided contact information and information about their products and granted permission to use their information. Any provided listing is not necessarily an endorsement of the company or its products. Companies listed here do not necessarily have gluten-free foods available.

As always, you should personally check the ingredients **every time** you purchase a product. You should contact the company that manufactures your favorite products, especially those with any questionable ingredients, every three to six months. Remember, "If in doubt, leave it out." (Information provided in this section was accurate at the time permission was granted.)

The next page shows an example of a letter to clarify or confirm the status of the foods you want to serve/eat.

Your address
Date

Dear Sir or Madam:

My child is on a medically required diet for the treatment of celiac disease
[or dermatitis herpetiformis]. He/she must avoid the gluten protein found
in wheat, rye, and barley. The gluten triggers an immune response, which
damages the lining of the small intestine.

I am interested in using your product [insert product name, e.g., X Brand
Ranch Salad Dressing]. The ingredient listing does not give adequate information for me to determine whether it is suitable for my child's medically
required diet. I need your assistance to determine whether he/she can safely
eat your product. Specifically, I need to know [insert—see examples below]:

> Examples:
> - The source of your "modified food starch."
> - Whether your "soy sauce solids" are derived from wheat.
> - What "natural flavorings" you use in your product.
> - The source of your "vegetable gum."
> - The inactive ingredients used in the medication, including those
>   ingredients used in the coatings and capsules.
> - The source of the "malt flavoring."
> - The source of the "caramel coloring."

Another source of gluten contamination is the secondary ingredients used
in the packaging and processing of some products. Since these secondary
ingredients are not listed on the packaging, I would greatly appreciate your
thoroughness in clarifying these substances in your product, if any.

Thank you for your efforts on my behalf.

Respectfully,
Your signature

American Pop Corn Company
P.O. Box 178
Sioux City, IA 51102
(712) 239-1232 (Mon.–Fri., 8 AM–5 PM CST)
Web site: www.jollytime.com
JOLLY TIME Pop Corn does not contain the gluten that comes from wheat, rye, oats, and barley. Therefore, people who are gluten intolerant can eat popcorn.

AriZona
(Ferolito Vultaggio & Sons)
5 Dakota Drive, Suite 205
Lake Success, NY 11042
(516) 812-0300 (9 AM–6 PM EST)
azbev@fuse.net
Products include iced teas, diet teas, punch and juice drinks, virgin cocktails, lemonades, sparkling sodas, isotonic sport drink, coffees, and snack foods.

Arm & Hammer Division
Church & Dwight Co., Inc
P.O. Box 1625
Horsham, PA 19044-6625
(800) 524-1328
Arm & Hammer® Baking Soda is 100 percent sodium bicarbonate and is free of gluten.

Beatrice Foods
Division of Beatrice Group, Inc.
4300 West 62nd Street
Indianapolis, IN 46268
(800) 988-7808 (8 AM–5 PM EST)
Products include Blue Bonnet spreads, Fleischman's margarine and spreads, Parkay spreads, Chiffon margarine, Move Over Butter spread, Touch of Butter spread, and Egg Beaters Real Egg Product.

Burger King
Consumer Information
P.O. Box 020783
Miami, FL 33102-0783
(305) 378-3535
Web site: www.burgerking.com
Look at the Burger King® Nutrition Guide, available at the restaurant, for information about our products.

Bush Brothers & Company
1016 East Weisgarber Road
Knoxville, TN 37909-2683
(865) 588-7685
All BUSH'S BEST products are gluten-free [at the time of publication] with the EXCEPTION of our BUSH'S BEST CHILI BEANS and BUSH'S CHILI MAGIC line. We do use cornstarch in some of our products. In order to ensure that a product is gluten-free, it is always possible to call our customer relations personnel.

Campbell Soup Company
World Headquarters
1 Campbell Place
Camden, NJ 08103-1799
(800) 257-8443
Web site: www.campbellsoup.com

Del Monte Foods
One Market
P.O. Box 193575
San Francisco, CA 94119-3575
(800) 543-3090 (8 AM–5 PM PST)
Web site: www.delmonte.com
     Gluten-free products include all canned/jarred fruits, all canned vegetables, all snack cups, tomatoes and tomato products, and all 100% fruit juices.

Dreyer's Grand Ice Cream
5929 College Ave.
Oakland, CA 94618
(510) 652-8187 (8 AM–5 PM PST)
Websites: www.dreyers.com
www.edys.com
www.icecream.com
     Products sold include Dreyer's Grand Ice Cream, Grand Light, No Sugar Added Ice Cream, Homemade Ice Cream, Fat Free/No Sugar Added Ice Cream, Frozen Yogurt, Fat Free Ice Cream, Sherbet, Fat Free Frozen Yogurt, Whole Fruit frozen fruit bars, and Whole Fruit Sorbet. Also Edy's Brand Products.

FritoLay, Inc.
Plano, TX 75024-4099
(800) 352-4477 (9 AM–4:30 PM, CST)

General Mills
P.O. Box 200
Minneapolis, MN 55440
(800) 328-1144; (800) 249-0562 (Mon.–Fri., 7:30 AM–5:30 PM CST)
Web site: www.generalmills.com
     Products include: Big G cereals, Betty Crocker products, Gold Medal flour, Robin Hood Flour, Bisquick, Nature Valley Granola, Gardetto's snacks, Bugles, Farmhouse Foods products, Pop Secret popcorn, Yoplait & Colombo yogurt, and Lloyd's Barbecued Meats. "We label our products with a separate 'contains' statement for the leading food allergens."

Gerber Products Company
560 Morris Avenue
Summit, NJ 07901-1312
(908) 598-7624 (9 AM–5 PM EST)
Web site: www.gerber.com

Gillian's Food Service
462 Proctor Avenue
Revere, MA 02151-5730
(781) 286-4095 (8 AM–4 PM EST)
FAX (781) 286-1933
Web site: www.GilliansFoods.com

Hillshire Farm & Kahn's
P.O. Box 25111
Cincinnati, OH 45225
(800) 328-2426 (8 AM–4:30 PM EST)
Web site: www.hillshirefarm.com

Hormel Foods Corporation
1 Hormel Place
Austin, MN 55912
(800) 523-4635 (7 AM–3:30 PM CST)
www.hormel.com

Idahoan Foods
Idaho Fresh-Pak, Inc.
P.O. Box 130
529 North 3500 East
Lewisville, ID 83431
(208) 754-4686 (8 AM–5 PM MST)
Web site: www.idahoan.com

"Idahoan Foods does not use any gluten-containing products in our processing, packaging containers, or package surfaces of our products. Some of our Idahoan® Potato products that could be used for gluten-free diets are Idahoan® Potato Flakes, REAL Complete Mashed potatoes, REAL Hash Browns, and Idahoan® Complete® Mix Mashed Potatoes. Also, our Idahoan® Augratin and Scalloped potatoes contain <0.01% protein from modified wheat or cornstarch."

Jack in the Box, Inc.
9330 Balboa Ave.
San Diego, CA 92123
(800) 955-5225 (Mon.–Fri., 8 AM–5:30 PM, PST)
Web site: www.jackinthebox.com

Nutritional information is available on our website.

KFC*
Web site: www.kfc.com

Kraft Foods, Inc.
(800) 323-0768
Web site: www.kraftfoods.com

Divisions include: Capri Sun, Maxwell House, Pizza Hut, and General Foods. The company is updating a list of gluten-free products. After this is finalized, contact them using the 800 number or web site listed above. "We suggest that consumers check the label every time they purchase a Kraft product in case the ingredients have changed."

Kroeger Herb Products
805 Walnut Street
Boulder, CO 80302
(800) 516-0690 (9 AM–5 PM, MST)
> Makers of "Totally Kids Nutrition" products.

Lawry's Foods, Inc.
Consumer Services
800 Sylvan Avenue
Englewood Cliffs, NJ 07632
(800) 745-9232
Web site: www.lawrys.com
> Products include spice blends, gravy mixes, seasoning blends, marinades, and salad dressings. Lawry's has an extensive list of gluten-free products too large to list here. Please contact them for a copy to be sent to you.

Long John Silver's Restaurants, Inc.
300 West Vine Street
P.O. Box 11988
Lexington, KY 40579-1988
(606) 543-6000 (8 AM–5 PM EST)
Web site: www.ljsilvers.com
> Items with no gluten-containing ingredients: corn, baked potato, green beans, coleslaw, side & garden salads, and all salad dressings.

Lundberg Family Farms
5370 Church Street
Richuale, CA 95974
(530) 882-4551 (8 AM–5 PM PST)
Web site: www.lundberg.com

Malt-O-Meal Company
Consumer Response
P.O. Box 631
Northfield, MN 55057
(800) 743-3029 (8 AM–4 PM CST)
Web site: www.malt-o-meal.com
> Malt-o-Meal has four gluten-free products: Malt-o-Meal Puffed Rice Cereal; Malt-o-Meal Corn Bursts Cereal; Malt-o-Meal Fruity Dyno-Bites® Cereal; Malt-o-Meal Cocoa Dyno-Bites® Cereal

McCormick & Co., Inc.
Consumer Affairs Department
211 Schilling Circle
Hunt Valley, MD 21031
(800) 632-5847
Web site: www.mccormick.com

McDonald's*
Web site: www.mcdonalds.com/countries/usa/food/index.html

Mead Johnson Nutritionals
2400 W. Lloyd Expressway
Evansville, IN 47721
(800) 222-9123 (Mon.–Fri., 7 AM–7 PM, CST; Sat., 8 AM–4:30 PM)
Web site: www.meadjohnson.com

Nabisco, Inc.
Consumer & Scientific Affairs
100 DeForest Avenue
P.O. Box 1911
East Hanover, NJ 07936-1911
800-NABISCO (800-633-4726) (10 AM–5 PM EST)
www.NABISCOWORLD.com

Northwest Natural Foods, Inc.
6644 Sexton Dr.
Olympia, WA 98502
(360) 866-9661 (Mon.–Fri., 8 AM–5 PM, PST)
    Makers of Salmon Medallions, Halibut Medallions, and Tuna Pesto Medallions.

Ocean Spray Cranberries, Inc.
One Ocean Spray Drive
Lakeville-Middleboro, MA 02349
(508) 946-1000

Ovaltine
P.O. Box 5329
Lakeworth, FL 33466-5329
(800) 442-0099

Pepsi-Cola Company
Consumer Relations Dept.
1 Pepsi Way
Somers, NY 10589
(800) 433-2652 (9 AM–6 PM, EST)

Pizza Hut*
Web site: www.pizzahut.com/more.asp

The Quaker Oats Company
P.O. Box 049003
Chicago, IL 60604-9003
(800) 694-7487 (8 AM–6 PM, CST)

Ralston Foods
Division of Ralcorp Holdings, Inc.
P.O. Box 618
St. Louis, MO 63188-0618
(800) 725-7866 (Mon.–Fri., 9 AM–4 PM, CST)
Web site: www.ralstonfoods.com

Red Star® Yeast & Products
A Division of Universal Foods Corporation
P.O. Box 737
Milwaukee, WI 53201
(800) 4-CELIAC (1-800-423-5422)
(414) 371-6755
Web site: www.redstaryeast.net
       Also has a free brochure of recipes entitled *New Gluten-Free Recipes for your Bread Machine from RED STAR® Yeast & Products.* Some of their recipes are used with permission in the *Breads* chapter.

Rice Select
P.O. Box 1305
Alvin, TX 77512
(800) 993-RICE
www.riceselect.com

Rising Sun Farms, Inc.
5126 S. Pacific Hwy.
Phoenix, OR 97535
(541) 535-8331 (8 AM–5 PM, PST)
www.risingsunfarms.com

S. Martinelli & Company
P.O. Box 1868
Watsonville, CA 95077
(800) 662-1868 (8 AM–12 PM; 1–5 PM, PST)
www.martinellis.com

Safeway Inc.
3540 Milleford Ct.
Pleasanton, CA 94588
(925) 467-3000 (8 AM–6 PM PST)
www.safeway.com

San-J International
2880 Sprouse Drive
Richmond, VA 23231
(804) 226-8333; (800) 446-5500 (8 AM–5 PM, EST)
Web site: www.san-j.com

Seneca Foods Corporation
3736 South Main Street
Marion, NY 14505
(315) 926-4284

Stash Tea Company
P.O. Box 910
Portland, OR 97207
(503) 684-4482 (8 AM–5 PM, PST)
Web site: www.stashtea.com
"All stash teas are gluten free with the exception of Genmai Rice. It contains brown rice."

Taco Bell*
Web site: www.tacobell.com

TCBY
425 W. Capitol Ave.
Suite 1200
Little Rock, AR 72201
(501) 688-8229 (8 AM–5 PM, CST)
Web site: www.tcby.com

Tofutti Brands, Inc.
50 Jackson Drive
Crawford, NJ 07016
(908) 272-2400 (9 AM–7 PM, EST)
Web site: www.tofutti.com
All items are dairy-free. The flavorings cannot be guaranteed to be gluten-free.

Weider Nutrition Int., Inc.
2002 South 5070 West
Salt Lake City, UT 84104
(800) 444-5200 (Mon.–Fri., 8 AM–5 PM, MST)
Web site: www.weider.com

---

* Asterisk indicates contact information about a company is in the public domain, but was not supplied by the company itself.

Organizations & Support Groups

*"The doctor of the future will give no medicine,
but will interest his patients in the care of the human body,
in diet, and in the cause and prevention of disease."*

—Thomas Edison

Allergies

Food Allergy & Anaphylaxis Network (FAAN)
10400 Eaton Place
Suite 107
Fairfax, VA 22030
(800) 929-4040
Web site: www.foodallergy.org

Parents of Allergic Children
P.O. Box 1808
Midlothian, VA 23113

Autism

Autism Services Center
605 9th Street, Prichard Building
P.O. Box 507
Huntington, WV 25710-0507
(304) 525-8014
FAX (304) 525-8026
Web site: www.autismservices.com

Autism Society of America
Director, Information and Referral Services
7910 Woodmont Avenue
Suite 300
Bethesda, MD 20814-3015
(800) 3AU-TISM; (301) 657-0881
FAX (301) 657-0869
Web site: www.autism-society.org

Autism Research Institute
4182 Adams Avenue
San Diego, CA 92116
FAX (619) 563-6840
Web site: www.autism.com

Center for the Study of Autism
P.O. Box 4538
Salem, OR 97302
Web site: www.autism.org

Celiac Disease

American Celiac Society/Dietary Support Coalition (ACS)
48 Musano Court
West Orange, NJ 07052
(973) 325-8837
E-mail: bentleac@umdnj.edu

Canadian Celiac Association
5170 Dixie Road, Suite 204
Mississauga, Ontario
L4W 1E3
(800) 363-7296; (905) 507-6208
FAX (905) 507-4673
Web site: www.celiac.ca

Celiac Disease Foundation (CDF)
13251 Ventura Blvd., Suite 1
Studio City, CA 91604
(818) 990-2354
FAX: (818) 990-2379
Web site: www.celiac.org

Celiac Sprue Association/USA, Inc. (CSA/USA)
P.O. Box 31700
Omaha, NE 68131-0700
(402) 558-0600
FAX: (402) 558-1347
Web site: www.csaceliacs.org

Coeliac Society of Australia
Web site: www.celiac.org.au

Coeliac Society of the United Kingdom
P.O. Box 220
High Wycome, Bucks HP 11 2HY
England, UK
(44) 494-437278
Web site: www.celiac.co.uk

Friends of Celiac Disease Research, Inc.
8832 North Port Washington Road, #204
Milwaukee, Wisconsin 53217
(414) 540-6679
FAX: (414) 540-0587
Web site: friendsofceliac.com

Gluten Intolerance Group
15110 10th Avenue SW, Suite A
Seattle, WA 98166
(206) 246-6652
FAX 206-246-6531
Web site: www.gluten.net

Down Syndrome

National Down Syndrome Congress
1370 Center Drive, Suite 102
Atlanta, GA 30338
(800) 232-6372
Web site: www.ndsccenter.org

National Down Syndrome Society
666 Broadway, 8th Floor
New York, NY 10012-2317
(800) 221-4602; (212) 460-9330
FAX: (212) 979-2873
Web site: www.ndss.org

Mental Health

Federation of Families for Children's Mental Health
1021 Prince Street
Alexandria, VA 22314-2971
(703) 684-7710
FAX: (703) 836-1040
Web site: www.ffcmh.org

National Institute of Mental Health
National Institutes of Health
Information Resources and Inquiries
6001 Executive Boulevard
Room 8184, MSC 9663
Bethesda, MD 20892-9663
(301) 443-4513 (Public Inquiries, 8:30 AM–5:00 PM)
FAX (301) 443-4279
 Web site: www.nimh.nih.gov

Other

American Autoimmune Related Diseases Association, Inc.
22100 Gratiot Avenue
Eastpointe
East Detroit, MI 48021-2227
(800) 598-4668
FAX (810) 776-3903
Web site: www.aarda.org

Recommended Reading

"Some books are to be tasted,
others are to be swallowed,
and some few to be chewed and digested."

—Francis Bacon

Fenster, Carol. *Special Diet Solutions: Healthy Cooking without Wheat, Gluten, Dairy, Eggs, Yeast, or Refined Sugar.* Littleton, CO: Savory Palate, 1997.

_____. *Special Diet Celebrations: No Wheat, Gluten, Dairy, or Eggs.* Littleton, CO: Savory Palate, 1999.

_____. *Wheat-Free Recipes and Menus.* Littleton, CO: Savory Palate, 1995.

Hagman, Bette. *The Gluten-Free Gourmet: Living Well without Wheat.* New York: Henry Holt, 2000.

_____. *The Gluten-Free Gourmet Bakes Bread: More than 200 Wheat-Free Recipes.* New York: Henry Holt, 1999.

_____. *The Gluten-Free Gourmet Cooks Fast and Healthy: Wheat-Free and Gluten-Free with No Fuss and Fat.* New York: Henry Holt, 1996.

_____. *The Gluten-Free Gourmet Dessert Cookbook.* New York: Henry Holt, 2002.

_____. *More from the Gluten-Free Gourmet: Delicious Dining without Wheat.* New York: Henry Holt, 1993.

Korn, Danna. *Kids with Celiac Disease: A Family Guide to Raising Happy, Healthy, Gluten-free Children.* Bethesda, MD: Woodbine House, 2001.

Lowell, Jax Peters. *Against the Grain: The Slightly Eccentric Guide to Living Well without Gluten or Wheat.* New York: Henry Holt, 1995.

Rapp, Doris. *Is This Your Child?* New York: Quill/William Morrow, 1991.

Reilly, Rebecca. *Great Gluten-Free Goodies.* Portland, ME: Rebecca's Kitchen, 1997.

Rottmann, Leon H. *On the Gluten-Free Condition: A Handbook for Celiac Patients and Their Families.* Omaha, NE: Celiac Sprue Association, 1998.

Sully's Living Without Magazine, Sully's Living Without, Inc., P.O. Box 2126, Northbrook, IL 60065. (847) 480-8810; www.livingwithout.com

Indexes

Recipe Index

G

Garfava flour, 29
Garlic Biscuits, 52
Garlic Toast, 64
Gelatin, unflavored, 28, 46
Ginger Snaps, Grain-Free, 220-21
Gingerbread Cut-Outs, 219
Glaze. *See* Icing
Gluten-Free Play Dough, 268-69
Graham Crackers. *See* Chocolate Graham
    Crackers; Grain-Free Honey Grahams
Grain-Free Cookies
  Grain-Free Ginger Snaps, 220-21
  Grain-Free Honey Grahams, 222-23
  Grain-Free Nut Butter Cookies, 224
Green Bean Amandine, 189
Green Beans with Cheese Sauce, 186.
Green Chili Casserole, 139
Ground beef. *See* Beef
Ground turkey. *See also* Poultry
  Ground Turkey Meatloaf, 141
  Ground Turkey Meatloaf Patties, 141
Guacamole, 251

H

Ham. *See* Pork
Ham Salad, 176
Hamburger. *See* Beef
Hamburger Buns, 65
Hamburger Casserole, Cheesy, 114
Herb Rice, 162
High altitude cooking, 289-92
Honey Barbecue Sauce, 111. *See also* Barbecue Sauce
Honey Grahams, Grain-Free, 222-23
Hot Dog Buns, 66
Hot Dogs, 252
Hot Tuna Tempties, 105

I

Icing. *See also* Cakes; Cookies; Old Fashioned
    Cake Doughnuts; Pies
  Almond Glaze, 213
  Chocolate Icing, 94-95
  Chocolate Sour Cream Frosting, 211
  Lemon Glaze, 213
  Lemon Icing, 94-95
  Maple Icing, 94-95
  Mocha Icing, 94-95
  Orange Glaze, 213
  Orange Icing, 94-95
  Powdered Sugar Glaze, 213, 244
  Sour Cream Frosting, 212, 259, 264
  White Frosting, 214, 259, 264
Individual-Size Pizza, 149-50
  Traditional Pizza Crust, 149-50
  Yeast-Free Bean Flour Pizza Crust, 151-52

Yeast-Free Individual Pizza Crust, 153-54
Ingredients
  common, 28
  questionable, 2-5
  specialty, 28-29
Italian Popcorn, 43

J

Juice. *See* Drinks.
Juicy Kool-Aid®, 39, 250-51, 253-54

K

Kielbasa and Rice, 117

L

Ladybugs, 40, 254
Lasagna, 118-19
LEGO Cake, 265
Lemon Bars, 225
Lemon Glaze, 213
Lemon Icing, 94-95
Lemon Yogurt Fruit Dressing, 180
Lima Beans. *See* Barbecue Butter Beans
Little Smokies, 252

M

Macaroni. *See* Pasta
Macaroni-N-Cheese, Baked, 156, 252
Macaroni Salad, 174
Maple Icing, 94-95
Markers, 272
Measuring. *See* Metric equivalents
Meat. *See* Beef; Fish; Pork; Poultry
Meatballs, Porcupine, 122, 253
Meatloaf. *See also* Beef; Poultry
  Ground Turkey Meatloaf, 141
  Ground Turkey Meatloaf Patties, 141
  Meatloaf Patties, 120
  Meaty Beef Meatloaf, 120
Metric equivalents, 287
Mexican Popcorn, 43
Microwave S'mores, 237
Milk-Free Bread
  Almond Bread, 58-59
  Apple Bread, 54-55
  Applesauce Bread, 54-55
  Milk-Free Cinnamon Nut Bread, 69-70
  Milk-Free Cinnamon Nut Rolls, 69-70
  Milk-Free Classic White Bread, 62-63
  Milk-Free Mock Rye Bread, 67-68
  Milk-Free Rice Tapioca Bread, 69-70, 253
  Milk-Free Sesame Bread, 71-72
  Milk-Free Whole Grain Brown Rice Bread, 73-74
  Zucchini Bread, 54-55
Milk-Free Pudding
  Milk-Free Banana Pudding, 235-36

Trail Mix, Peanut-Free, 42
troubleshooting, 279-86
Tuna. *See* Fish
Tuna Casserole, 108
Tuna Salad, 176
Turkey. *See* Poultry
Turnips with Cheese Sauce, 186.

U
Unflavored gelatin, 28, 46

V
Vanilla Frosting. *See* White Frosting
Vanilla Pudding, Creamy, 235-36. *See also*
    Milk-Free Vanilla Pudding
Vegetable Dip, Dilly, 179

W
Waffles, 99
Watercolor Paints, 272
Whipping Cream, Mock, 239
White Bread, Classic, 62-63
White Cake, Classic, 206
White Frosting, 214, 259, 264
Whole Grain Brown Rice Bread, 73-74. *See also*
    Milk-Free Whole Grain Brown Rice Bread
Winter Soup, 198

X
Xanthan gum, 29

Y
Yams. *See* Baked Potatoes
Yeast breads, 57-74
Yeast-Free
    Yeast-Free Bean Flour Individual Pizza Crust,
        151-52
    Yeast-Free Bean Flour Pizza Crust, 151-52
    Yeast-Free Individual Pizza Crust, 153-54

Z
Zucchini Bread, 54-55

EZ Easy Recipes Index

Refer to the Recipe Index (pp. 318-25) for page numbers.

Almond Glaze
Apple Fritters
Apple Salad
Baked French Fries
Baked Garlic Parmesan Fries
Baked Macaroni-N-Cheese
Baked Potato Skins
Baked Potatoes
Banana Muffins
Banana Nut Muffins
Barbecue Chicken Nuggets
Barbecue Sauce
Biscuits Supreme
Blackberry Muffins
Blueberry Muffins
Breakfast Muffins
Broccoli with Cheese Sauce
Brown Rice Crackers
Brown Rice Pilaf
Buggy Bananas
Busy Day Cake
Busy Day Chocolate Cake
Busy Day Pineapple Upside Down Cake
Busy Day Spiced Cake
Buttered Popcorn
Buttermilk Biscuits
Buttermilk Dressing
Buttermilk Pancakes
Caramel Corn
Carrot Cake
Cheesy Tortillas
Chicken and Alfredo Sauce
Chicken and Rice Soup
Chicken Biscuit Surprise
Chicken Noodle Soup
Chicken Nuggets
Chicken Salad
Chicken Vegetable Soup
Chicken with Dijon Sauce
Chili with Beans
Chocolate Candy Cookies
Chocolate Chip Cookies
Chocolate Chip Muffins
Chocolate Sour Cream Frosting
Classic White Cake
Corn Bread
Corn Muffins
Cowboy Coffee Cake

Cranberry Muffins
Cream Cheese Fruit Dressing
Cream of Chicken Soup
Cream of Tomato Soup
Creamy Coleslaw
Creamy Green Bean Casserole
Creamy Pasta Salad
Creamy Potato Salad
Crustless Quiche
Curried Rice Mix
Devil's Food Cake
Deviled Eggs
Dilly Vegetable Dip
Easy Baked Beans
Egg Salad
Egg-Free Rice Pudding
Fruitful Party Punch
Fudge Brownies
Garlic Biscuits
Garlic Toast
Grain-Free Ginger Snaps
Green Bean Amandine
Ground Turkey Metloaf
Ham Salad
Herb Rice
Honey Barbecue Sauce
Hot Tuna Tempties
Italian Popcorn
Juicy Kool-Aid®
Kielbasa and Rice
Ladybugs
Lemon Glaze
Lemon Yogurt Fruit Dressing
Macaroni Salad
Meaty Beef Meatloaf
Mexican Popcorn
Microwave S'mores
Mini Pizzas
Mock Whipping Cream
Nachos
Noodles in Alfredo Sauce
One Skillet Beef Stroganoff
Orange Glaze
Parmesan Popcorn
Peanut-Free Trail Mix
Pizza Sauce
Popcorn
Porcupine Meatballs

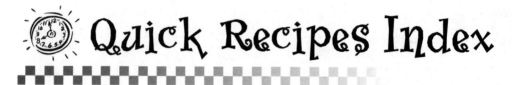

Quick Recipes Index

Refer to the Recipe Index (pp. 318-25) for page numbers.

Finger-Food Recipes Index

Refer to the Recipe Index (pp. 318-25) for page numbers.

Subject Index

■■■■■■■■■■■■■■■■■■■■■■■

About the Author

Sheri L. Sanderson is the mother of three children, including one with gluten sensitivities and autism. Her cookbook is the result of personal need—wanting to offer her family gluten-free meals that look and taste just as good as those she made before the change in diet. She lives with her family in San Marcos, California.